THE PERFECT ALKALINE DIET GUIDE FOR BEGINNERS

Increase Your Energy and Prevent
Diabetes and Other Diseases

Table of Contents

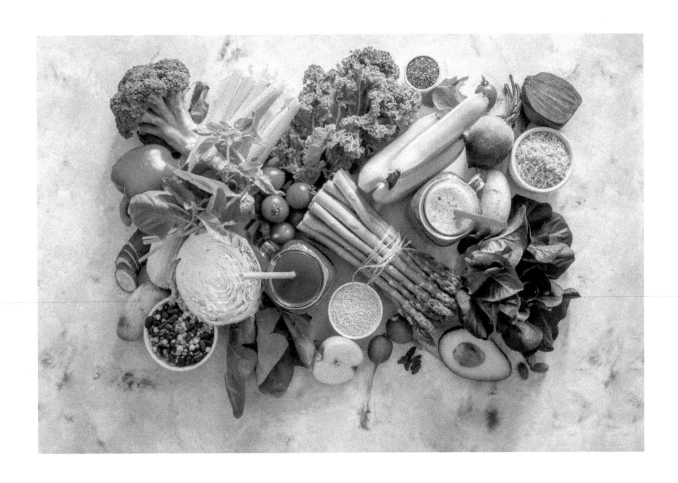

Introduction

In this book, you will learn all of the healing secrets of Dr. Sebi and how they can help you to improve your health.

This is why in this book, we are going to take a closer look at some cogent points made by Dr. Sebi. The Honduran herbalist, Dr. Sebi is well revered for positively changing the lives of many around the world with his herbal knowledge. These so-called changes were made possible by an alkaline diet which he tagged "African Bio-Electric Cell Food Therapy."

Choosing alkaline foods is the only way to live and lose extra pounds for healthy living.

It's believed to rebuild your cells by removing radioactive waste by alkalizing the blood. Dr. Sebi was not a doctor, considering his position, and did not possess a Ph.D.

He developed this diet for those seeking to treat or avoid diseases and enhance their general wellbeing without focusing on traditional Western medication.

Dr. Sebi's Diet is not approved by official sources and no scientific evidence shows that medical conditions can be prevented or treated using this method.

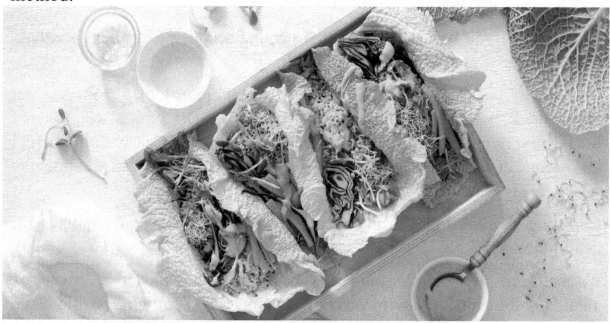

Who Is Dr. Sebi?

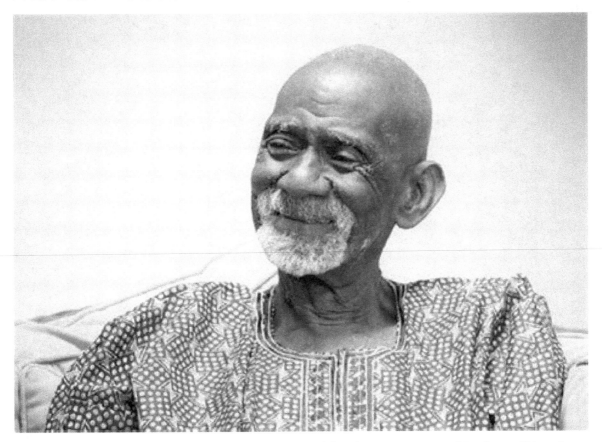

The man behind the Dr. Sebi Diet is Alfredo Bowman. He is a Honduran self-proclaimed herbalist and healer who used food to improve health. Although he is already deceased, he has a number of followers in the 21st century. Because of his holistic approach, he claimed to cure many kinds of diseases using herbs and a strict vegan diet. He set up a treatment center in his home country before moving to New York City, where he continued his practice and extended his clienteles to Michael Jackson, John Travolta, Eddie Murphy, and Steven Seagal, to name a few.

Although he called himself Dr. Sebi, he did not hold any medical nor Ph.D. degree. Moreover, the diet has claimed to cure different conditions such as sickle-cell anemia, lupus, leukemia, and HIV-AIDS. This led to a lot of issues, particularly that he was practicing medicine without a license and his exorbitant claims. While he was charged for practicing without a license, he was acquitted in the early 1990s due to a lack of evidence. However, he was instructed to stop making claims that his diet can treat HIV-AIDS. While there are controversies that surround his name, there are so many benefits of his alkaline vegan diet that it is still popular even to this date.

Alkaline Diet

Consuming an alkaline diet promotes good health and eating more helps fight disease while acidic food promotes it. Acid-alkaline homeostasis is the pH level that the human body maintains. Food's tendency to form acidity or alkalinity has no role to play with the food's pH.

For example, lemons' final product after ingestion and assimilation is very alkaline, but the nature of the fruits themselves is acidic. Hence, lemons are alkaline. Likewise, the meat's flavor is alkaline, but its final product is an acidic residue.

Throwing fruits and vegetables into the mix with their health benefits and phytochemicals is necessary to stay active, healthy, and energetic.

It is highly recommended that 80% of what you eat be composed of alkaline foods and 20% acid-forming foods. While over 60% of the food you consume should be alkaline-producing food, and less than 40% of the food consumed should be acid-forming food for maintaining health.

The pH is highly contained in all biological fluids and tissues within a very close range.

What Exactly Is the Alkaline Diet?

The alkaline diet is based on considering that a diet rich in acidic foods disturbs the body's acid-base balance, promoting the loss of essential minerals, such as calcium and magnesium, in the bones. Such alterations would favor the appearance of chronic mild acidosis, which in turn would be a predisposing factor for some diseases and a sense of general malaise.

The alkaline diet recommends consuming 70–80% of alkaline foods and 20–30% of acidic foods every day. This food model is closer to that followed by man until discovering agriculture than the current one.

Cells, tissues, organs, and systems work best when the pH is essential. The human body is made to be slightly alkaline, with a pH range from 7.1 to 7.5 —with an optimal value between 7.39 and 7.41. Normal physiological activities, as well as the intake of some foods, instead determine an acidic environment.

How to bring our body back to the right pH? Easy, just feed properly, preferring alkaline foods rich in potassium, magnesium, and calcium. Keep in mind that a diet that abounds in meat and industrial products is the most acidifying one and should therefore be avoided (or in any case severely reduced) in favor of a plant-based diet. The right daily balance is given by the intake of 70% of essential foods, 20% of acidic foods, and 10% of neutral foods.

An acidic environment predisposes to the formation of inflammation, the lowering of the immune defenses, and in general, to a state of psychophysical discomfort and cellular aging.

Factors Making Diets Alkaline

Alkaline foods are mainly of vegetable origin and rich in minerals and vitamins. Here is a list of alkaline and beneficial foods:

- **Vegetables:** mostly green leafy vegetables (spinach, chard, broccoli, cauliflower, and celery), cucumbers, and onions; the tubers are also excellent (carrots, pumpkins, potatoes).

- **Dried fruits:** especially almonds.

- **Whole grains:** preferably gluten-free (millet, amaranth, brown rice, red rice, black rice, buckwheat, and quinoa). When we realize that our body tends to acidosis, we can stock up on essential minerals by consuming the following alkalizing superfoods.

- **Umeboshi plum:** a particular apricot fermented in brine in miso leaves.

- **Seaweed:** kombu, wakame, spirulina, hiziki, arame, kelp, and dulse.

Aloe juice, oil and flax seeds, Lorraine, sprouts, kuzu, turmeric, ginger.

Since the diet is based on the pH of foods, some versions are very harsh, while others, despite their slightly acidic pH, manage to be implemented while also allowing cereals and their health benefits.

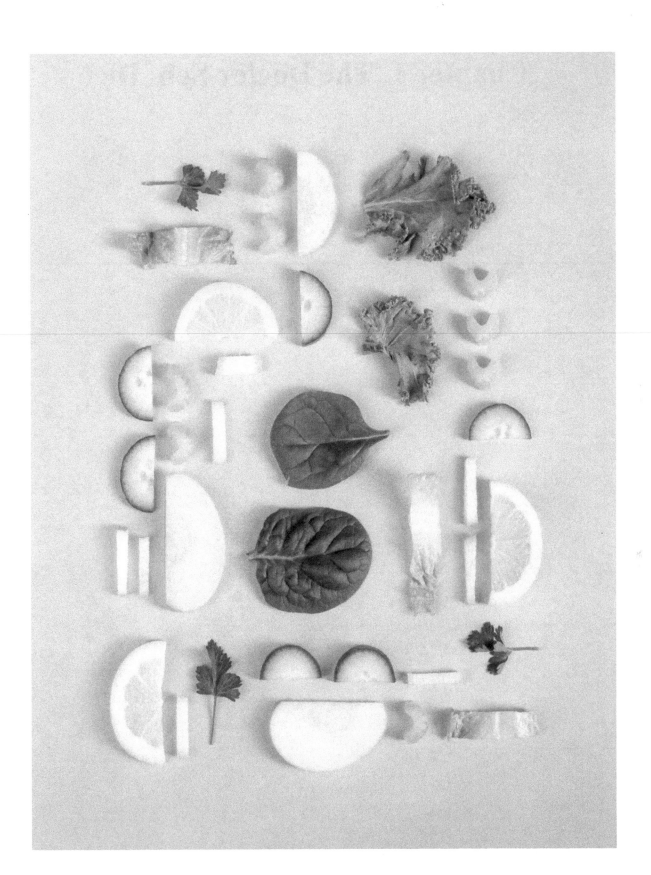

Chapter 1. The Doctor Sebi Diet

What Is the Doctor Sebi Diet?

Dr. Sebi believed that acidity and mucus could cause different types of diseases. For instance, the buildup of mucus in the lungs can lead to pneumonia. He noted that eating certain types of food, and avoiding others like the plague, can help detoxify the body. It can also bring the body to an alkaline state that can reduce the risk of developing many types of diseases. By turning the blood alkaline, the cells can be rejuvenated and can easily eliminate toxins out. Moreover, he argues that diseases cannot exist in an environment that is alkaline. His principle of making the body more alkaline is what other plant-based diets are banking on.

This particular diet relies on eating a list of approved foods as well as the intake of certain types of supplements. For the body to heal itself, Dr. Sebi noted that this diet should be followed consistently for the rest of your life.

The Dr. Sebi Diet is plant-based, but unlike other plant-based diets, there are some differences in this diet compared to the plant-based diet in general. Here is a compiled list of what differentiates the Dr. Sebi Diet from a plant-based diet.

No Processed Foods

Tofu, veggie burgers, textured vegetable protein, canned fruits, canned vegetables, oil, soy sauce, and other condiments are considered processed. The Dr. Sebi Diet encourages dieters to consume food that is unadulterated. Some plant-based diets still allow the consumption of processed foods, as long as they are made from plant-based ingredients.

No Wheat Products Allowed

Under this diet regimen, you are not allowed to consume wheat and wheat products such as bread, biscuits, and others as they are not naturally grown grains. Naturally grown grains include amaranth seeds, wild rice, and triticale, to name a few.

The Need to Adhere to the Food List

In general, plant-based diets are not so restrictive when it comes to the food that dieters are allowed to eat (unless you are specifically following a strict plant-based regimen such as the plant-based keto diet). However, the Dr.

Sebi Diet requires dieters to only eat foods that are listed in the nutritional guide.

Drink One (1) Gallon of Water Daily

Water is the most hydrating liquid on the planet. The Dr. Sebi Diet requires dieters to consume 1 gallon of water daily or more. Moreover, tea and coffee should be avoided as these drinks are highly acidic.

Taking Dr. Sebi's Supplements

If you are taking any medications for a particular health condition, this particular diet regimen will require you to consume proprietary supplements an hour before taking your medication.

What Was the Diet Based on?

He believed that the diseases inside our body are caused by the buildup of mucus in different organs—like if the heart had a buildup of mucus, it leads to heart disease, and if it is in excess in the pancreas, it causes diabetes. He also claimed that diseases thrive in acidic environments and die in an alkaline environment. He said that the diet would restore the body's original healthy start if we strictly follow it and consume the mixtures/supplements that he originally made. The body will then be cleansed and detoxified of harmful substances. Natural foods mentioned in this diet are high in alkalinity, and it raises the body pH, so according to Alfredo's theories, they can heal the body by creating an alkaline environment internally.

The diet is made up of lists of different vegetables, fruits, seeds, grains, nuts, and oils, with no addition of animal-sourced food. That is why the diet can also be considered a vegan diet. However, it is even more restrictive than that as some vegetables, grains, and fruits are banned from being consumed. For example, you are not permitted to eat seedless fruits in this diet. Also, to get the maximum and continuous benefit, Dr. Sebi says to follow this diet for the entirety of your life, which makes the diet even more strict and restrictive.

Dr. Sebi's Teachings and Methods

Dr. Sebi proposed that the body is in the state of becoming susceptible to contracting diseases when the level of toxins and mucus accumulation increases. He argued that people that are suffering from different diseases and those that are interested in preventing them should always eat an alkaline diet, bearing in mind that when the body removes the increased amount of acidic substances and mucus, it becomes free from infections.

He also suggested that cleansing and detoxification of the body is an essential and significant tool necessary in dealing with any form of the disease in the body. Detoxification of the body assists in the elimination of mucus accumulated in the liver, lungs, and many other body organs and also helps in the removal of excess acidic substances, thereby making the body free from disease-causing diseases.

Dr. Sebi also made use of herbs that are important in re-energizing and revitalizing the body. The organs of the body function properly when there is an improvement in your health, and this indicates that your body is void of diseases.

Some Disadvantages of Doctor Sebi Diet You Must Know

The alkaline diet by Dr. Sebi has a lot of disadvantages too. The following is a list of them:

- **Highly restrictive:** The diet's main con is that it hinders businesses that specialize in foods such as wheat, animal products, lentils, beans, and many other varieties of fruits and vegetables.

  The diet only allows specific fruit forms. An example is consuming plum or cherry tomatoes but no other forms like the Roma or beefsteak tomatoes. As the diet harshly criticizes ingredients that are not found in nutrition manuals, one can develop a negative attitude towards food. You will realize that following the diet is not always fun.

  Lastly, the weight-loss plan can encourage some bad behaviors and the use of supplements. The supplements are usually not the best source of calories. As a result, one ends up having poor styles of consuming foods.

- **Absence of proteins and other important vitamins:** Listed ingredients in the diet plan of Dr. Sebi can also act as good sources of vitamins. Nonetheless, not the certified foods can be the source of proteins, important nutrients for skin and pore structure, hormone, and enzyme production, and muscle boom. The only certified foods that have the proteins mentioned are hemp seeds, walnuts, Brazil nuts, and sesame seeds.

  To obtain the daily required proteins, you need to consume large amounts of the doctor's ingredients. The ingredients have a high concentration of nutrients like potassium, nutrients C and E, beta, and carotene. They have a low concentration of ingredients like iron, omega-3, vitamins B12 and D, and calcium.

Chapter 2. The Dr. Sebi Diet and Weight Loss

Weight Loss and Good Health

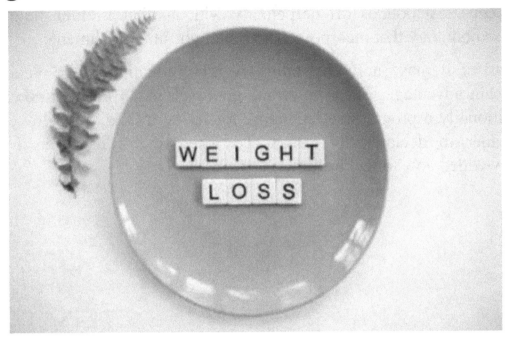

Lose weight! Look good! Increase energy! This section of the book will show you how it's done. Not alone, it will also show you how to change your life for the better. Thousands of famous and low profile men in history have followed its teachings and methods for decades. Most of you will have heard people with testimony saying it's the most effective weight loss program they've tried ever. Yes, it is! They've been through the weight-loss wars and conquered with this legend approached. List them and I tell it you've probably attempted it, regardless of whether it's a low-fat diet, a food-combining diet, the grapefruit diet, fluid diets, or other.

You've figured out how to check calories, in any case with no achievement. Regardless of whether you shed pounds, you were regularly ravenous and consistently felt denied. At that point when you returned to your old method of eating, those pounds crawled back, periodically joined by a couple of something else. If this scenario sounds very natural, I have an answer that will help end the round of yo-yo counting calories for the last time. All things being equal, I'll assist you with embracing a lasting method of eating that:

- Let's get in shape without counting calories.
- Make you feel and look better.

- Naturally re-stimulates you.

- Keeps lost pounds off perpetually with another lifetime nourishing methodology that incorporates rich, delightful nourishments.

Be that as it may, notwithstanding weight reduction, there is a more significant advantage: The wholesome approach you'll find out about here is additionally a progressive technique for living a long, solid life. I need my reader to declare: "I realized I'd lose weight; however, I never acknowledged how to feel healthier."

Changing Your Mindset

Have you gotten an idea up with the possibility that to lose weight and feel great you need to adopt a low-fat diet? Assuming this is the case, the standards and approach I'm going to outline for you might appear counterintuitive but will be very effective and outstanding. In the decade's years back when Dr. Sebi published his first research and claim, then a new logical and scientific approach has been led, conducted, and published that shows that a controlled starch healthful methodology is better for you—and for your body—than low fat, high-starch nourishing methodology. But let quit wasting time. Here are three inquiries you ought to present yourself directly: Is this safe? Is this healthfully solid? Will I keep the weight off once I lose it?

- Safe? Indeed, and there is a lot of hard science to back that up. Truth be told, various investigations directed in the previous years show that a controlled sugar dietary methodology improves the clinical boundaries influencing coronary illness and different diseases while not causing harm to your liver, kidneys, or bone structure.

- Healthfully solid? Truly, an individual after the regular menu and eating nourishments containing only 20 grams of carbohydrates meets or surpasses the day by day recommended amount of most vitamins, nutrients, and minerals. As you move through the phase of Dr. Sebi, you get much more. What's more, not as indicated by me but accepted by world well know organization and used by most of the practicing nutritionists.

- Keep off all the shed pounds? Nothing could be all the more obvious. Whenever you've seen the outcomes and conceded to great wellbeing, you'll understand that it's a lot simpler than you ever suspected conceivable. In view of the sorts of nourishments that are essential, it's really conceivable to roll out an improvement in the manner joyfully you eat (and look and feel) for good.

The Four Principle of Dr. Sebi Nutritional Approach to Weight Loss

Following the Dr. Sebi Nutritional Approach for weight, you will achieve four things:

- **You will get in shape:** it's hard not to. Either male or female who follow Dr. Sebi's way to deal with weight reduction promptly take off pounds and inches. For the little numbers who have a really no-nonsense metabolic protection from weight reduction, subsequent sections will broadly expand on the best way to defeat the hindrances that forestall a fruitful result. Streamlining body weight is an essential component of any wellbeing focused program in light of the fact that, all around, being essentially overweight is a marker of potential medical conditions, presently or later on. At the point when you've taken the pounds off, you'll see the advantages, and they will be definitely more than only corrective.

- **You will keep up your weight reduction:** this is the place where Dr. Sebi Nutritional Approach leaves most different weight control plans in the dust. Pretty much every accomplished calorie counter has started eating less, buckled down, lost a ton of pounds, and restored them all in a couple of months or maybe a year. This is typical because of the normal result of low-fat/low-calorie counts calories hunger. Although numerous individuals can endure hunger for some time, not many can endure it for a lifetime. Hardship is unpleasant. When the organic hole among yearning and satisfaction becomes excessively enormous, the bounce-back can be incredibly fast just as tragic and mortifying. However, that is the issue of diets that confine amounts. This program of approach won't acknowledge hunger as a lifestyle. The arrangement incorporates nourishments with enough fat and protein, so hunger isn't the enormous issue it is on other weight reduction plans. Be that as it may, it actually permits calorie counters to keep up a sound load for a lifetime.

- **You will accomplish great wellbeing:** the change is astounding. Doing Dr. Sebi, you meet your wholesome needs by eating tasty, sound, filling nourishments and dodging the sugar and carbs that lousy nourishment is stacked with. Subsequently, you become not so much drained but rather more vivacious, not only in light of the weight reduction but since the physical results of really useless glucose and insulin digestion are turned around. Secondly, individuals begin feeling great even before they arrive at their objective weight. When they surrender the calamitous American eating regimen of refined sugars for entire, crude food, they begin to live once more.

- **You will lay the perpetual foundation for infection counteraction:** this will transform you, which, in all honesty, is much more significant than looking great on the seashore the following summer. By following an individualized controlled carbohydrate dietary methodology that outcomes in lower insulin creation, individuals at high danger for persistent sicknesses, for example, cardiovascular illness, hypertension, and diabetes, will see a stamped improvement in their 15 clinical measures.

Why the Dr. Sebi Nutritional Approach?

The obvious fact is that millions of individuals don't eat the kinds of nourishments that are steady healthy metabolism. Humanity isn't equipped to deal with a bounty of refined sugars. Getting more fit doesn't involve tallying calories, it involves eating food your body can deal with. Let me place a couple of realities on the table, all of which we will investigate all through the rest of this book:

- Most obesity came into play when the body's digestion or metabolism cycle by which it transforms food into energy isn't functioning accurately. The more overweight an individual is, the more certain is the presence of metabolic unsettling influence.

- The foundation of the metabolic aggravation in heftiness doesn't have to do with the fat you eat, it has to do with eating an excessive amount of carbohydrate, which prompts metabolic issues, for example, insulin obstruction and hyper insulin. Furthermore, these metabolic issues are legitimately identified with your overall wellbeing picture and your probability of being misled by executioners such as diabetes, coronary illness, heart disease, and stroke. Additionally, high insulin levels have been related to a higher rate of diabetes.

- The metabolic effect also sources from excess insulin produced in the body which can be circumvented by a controlled sugary diet. Avoid the foods that cause you to be fat by controlling your intake of refined carbohydrates.

- This metabolic adjustment is striking to such an extent that some of us will have the option to lose weight by eating a higher number of calories than you've been eating on diets top-heavy unbalanced in sugars.

- Diets high in sugars are correctly what most overweight individuals don't require and can't turn out to be forever slim on. Low-fat weight control plans are, by their very nature, quite often rich-carbohydrate diets less and welcome on the very issues that they were expected to shield us from.

- Our pandemics of diabetes, coronary illness, and hypertension are to a great extent the adamant effects of our overconsumption of refined starches and its association with hyperinsulinism.

Different Kinds of Foods

Protein is a complex chain of amino acids, it's the fundamental structure block of life and basic to pretty much every synthetic response in the human body. Food wealthy in protein incorporates meat, fish, fowl, eggs (the greater part of which contain basically no carbohydrates), and cheese, nuts, and seeds. Numerous vegetables are additionally all around provided. However, dissimilar to other animal foods, don't contain all the fundamental amino acids.

Fat gives glycerol and basic unsaturated fat called fatty acids, which the body can't produce on its own. Fat is found in fish, fowl, meat, dairy items, and the oils got from nuts and seeds and a couple of vegetables, for example, avocados. Oils separated from these nourishments signify 100% fat and contain no carbohydrates.

Carbohydrate incorporates sugars and starches that are chains of sugar particles. Despite the fact that carbohydrate gives the snappiest source of energy, we eat substantially more of it, by a wide margin, than our body should be healthy. Vegetables do contain a few starches; however, they likewise contain a wide and wondrous variety of nutrients and minerals. Notwithstanding, you can eat many vegetables with high groupings of useful supplements and still control your junk. Then again, starches, for example, those in sugar and white flour contain practically nothing that your body needs in large quantities.

What Are We to Do?

If you need to be weight-smart and health-wise, you can't eat as I've portrayed. But you can eat the natural, fruit and vegetable nourishments as described by Dr. Sebi. Nor do you need to eat like a bunny; you can eat like a person. You can appreciate fish, sheep, steak and lobster, nuts and berries, eggs, and spread alongside a magnificent assortment of a plate of mixed greens, a variety of salad, and different vegetables.

What Do You Eat?

Do you accept that a man can go from gaining 0.5 pound seven days, a week to losing 3.9 pounds seven days without altogether modifying the number of calories he consumes? Let me tell you about Harry Clark. I need you to give close consideration to his story and make an effort not to offer disbelief to incredulity, on the grounds that these outcomes are genuine. Harry Clark, the 40-year-old director of a lumberyard, came to me with a heart arrhythmia and a frantic weight issue. He had been chubby even as a kid, yet now things were worse and out of hand. A couple of years prior, he had gone to a low-fat eating regimen focus and had figured out how to drop from 245 to 185 pounds, sounds great. Yet, in a little while, Harry had recovered everything with an additional profit of another 35 pounds.

Believe it or not, when Harry came to see me, he weighed in at 280 on a five-foot six-and-a-half-inch outline. In the past 35 months, eating a generally bland, low-fat diet of around 2,100 calories every day, he had increased 70 pounds, precisely 2 pounds per month. Harry began Dr. Sebi's Diet, radically restricting his consumption of carbohydrates while eating unreservedly of meat, fish, fowl, and eggs. Harry was told he could eat as much as he expected to feel fulfilled. The carbohydrate level was strikingly like what he had been eating on his past eating regimen. A quarter of a year into his new routine, he had lost 50.5 pounds (just about 4 pounds every week), and afterward kept on losing at a consistent 3 pounds' week by week. His heart manifestations disappeared, his absolute cholesterol level dropped from a mid-range 207 to a significantly lower 134 and his fatty went from 134 to 31.

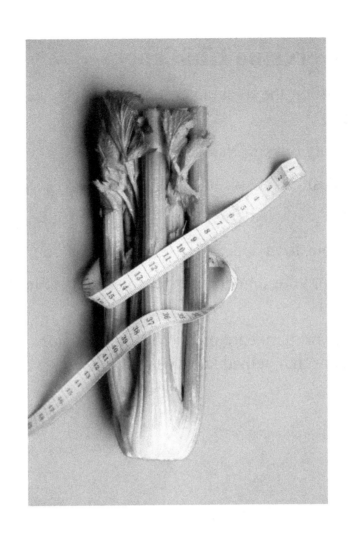

How to Overcome Challenges

- Get directly in the track again on the off chance that you sporadically "tumble off."

- Stop pigging out surprisingly fast.

- Manage desires for sweets and starches.

- Guarantee that what you lose is fat and not fit body tissue.

- Change your food decisions as indicated by your own metabolism.

- Supplement your dinners with vita nutrients to help conquer metabolic obstruction.

- With your primary care physician's supervision, wipe out specific medications that helped keep your obesity.

How to Get Healthy

- Defeat diet-related conditions, for example, unstable blood glucose, yeast diseases, and food bigotries.

- Dodge the wellbeing calamity of hyperinsulinism.

- Improve your energy level, which will make practice simpler.

- Locate the privilege vita nutrients to supplement the nourishments you eat for complete nutrition.

- Bring down your cholesterol and fatty substance levels and improve your other blood science esteems.

- Address the ailments particularly diabetes, coronary illness, and high blood pressure so frequently connected with obesity.

How to Deal With the Day-to-Day Issues

- Explore grocery store aisles to discover controlled junks, low-sugar nourishments.

- Eat out easily in exquisite eateries or even cheap food chains.

- Attend dinner gatherings without trading off your health improvement plan or blaming your hosts.

- Clarify your better approach to eating to love ones.

- Take some time off or go to uncommon capacities without cheating.

- Eat serenely with those whose style of eating remains not the same as yours.

What to Eat and How to Control Your Weight Gain

- Exercise is beneficial for you, and it will enable you to lose. Besides, it makes you burn calories; however, it quickens your metabolism, speeding up with which each other aspect of a weight loss program works and keeps you headed for better wellbeing.

- Now we briefly discuss the meal plans according to Dr. Sebi. Follow his menu for the first week, and then repeat it for another week.

Chapter 3. Effective, Regenerating, and Quick-Acting Strategies

Herbal Medicine

Herbal medicine is the expertise, techniques, and procedures centered on the philosophies, values, and interactions indigenous to various societies, utilized in the health preservation and health prevention, evaluation, enhancement, or cure of the mental and physical disorder.

Traditional medicine has several distinct structures, and the theory and each activity are regulated by the environment, different conditions, and geographical location of the area where it is evolved. Generally, regardless of the underlying ailment or illness by which the patient suffers, the emphasis is on the general health of the person, and the usage of the herb is a central aspect of many conventional medicine programs.

A significant representation of how classical and acquired information is implemented through a systematic approach to present-day medical care has been traditional Chinese medicine (TCM). TCM has over 3,000 years of history. The book "The Devine Farmer's Classic of Herbalism" was composed in China around 2,000 years back, and it is the world's oldest documented herbal text. However, the recorded and methodically gathered herbal knowledge has evolved into numerous herbal pharmacopeias, and there are several monographs on herbs individually.

Treatment and diagnosis, represented in light of the combination of ying-yang, are centered on a balanced perception of the disease and the effects of the disease. Ying portrays femininity, earth, and ice, while the sky, masculinity, and heat are depicted by yang. Ying and yang's acts impact the relationships of the 5 elements that make up the world: wood, water, metal, earth, and fire. TCM practitioners strive to regulate the degrees of yang and yin across 12 meridians that carry and guide energies (Qi) via a body. TCM is a rising procedure worldwide, and it is used both to improve wellbeing and to avoid and prevent disease. TCM contains several activities, but traditional remedies and natural elements are a crucial feature.

In some regions of the planet, health treatment has been revolutionized over the last 100 years by the invention and industrial manufacturing of chemically manufactured medicines. However, in developed countries, significant parts of the community also depend on conventional practitioners and natural remedies for the primary treatment.

Up to 90% of the people in Africa and 70% in India rely on traditional medication to treat their medical needs. Conventional medicine, in China, contributes to around 40% of all provided health care, and more than 90% of public hospitals have traditional medicine units. However, the usage of herbal remedies is not restricted to emerging nations, and the general interest in herbal remedies has significantly expanded in developed countries during the past two decades, with the increasing use of ethnobotanicals.

The most popular motives for utilizing natural medications are that they are more accessible, more generally correlates to the patient's lifestyle, allays fears regarding the harmful consequences of artificial (synthetic) drugs, fulfills a need for more customized healthcare facilitates a more comprehensive community approach to health records. The main application of herbal medications is the promotion of human health and therapy of chronic diseases and prevent life-threatening disorders. However, the use of natural remedies grows as current therapy is inadequate in clinical management, for example, in advanced tumors and modern contagious diseases. In comparison, natural drugs are commonly accepted, not poisonous, and are safe healthy.

Regardless of whether a person needs it, herbal medicine offers an essential health care commodity, whether individuals have financial or physical exposure to allopathic medication and is a growing worldwide market. Herbs are currently used to cure chronic and severe illnesses and different disorders and issues, such as heart disease, prostate disorders, obesity, asthma, anxiety, and improve immunity. Traditional natural remedies played a leading key role in the technique for controlling and curing SARS (Severe Acute Respiratory Syndrome) in China in 2003.

A conventional herbal medication, the African flower, is being used in Africa for ages to manage HIV-related symptoms. Natural medicines are still trendy in Europe. France and Germany, leading overall purchases by European countries, herbal extracts or teas, and essential oils may be found in pharmacy selling prescription medications in most developed countries.

Herbs and seeds, including whole herbs, teas, syrups, lavender oil, ointments, salves, rubbers, tablets, and capsules comprising a powdered type dry extract of a raw herb form, may be manufactured and may be taken in numerous ways and styles. Plant and herb extracts differ and include vinegar (extracts of acetic acid), alcoholic extracts, hot water extracts (tisanes), long boiling extracts, generally bark, and roots (decoctions), and cold plant infusions. There is a little specification, and an herbal product's ingredients mostly differ significantly across batches and manufacturers.

Plant species are abundant with a diversity of substances. Most are secondary plant metabolites that contain aromatic compounds, which are mostly phenols or variants of phenols supplemented with oxygen, like tannins. Many of those substances are antioxidants.

Herbal Treatment for Aging

In several developing nations, life expectancy rose, in the early 1950s, from about 41 years to about 80. Consequently, the proportion of the aged among our communities (sixty-five years and over) is growing. The greying of our societies carries a growing burden of illness and dependence correlated with chronic aging. Aging is linked with a gradual deterioration in neurological activity and an enhanced risk of death, coronary disease, hypertension, diabetes mellitus, dementia, osteoporosis, etc. Factors in lifestyle such as exercise or diet play a significant role in assessing the length and quality of healthy life and even treating infectious diseases. There is not any apparent reason for aging, though multiple hypotheses of aging have been proposed over the years.

Genetic influences are undeniably significant, but of all the metabolic explanations of aging, the most widely supported theory is the oxidative stress hypothesis (Beckman and Ames 1998; Harman 1992). This hypothesis postulates that aging is triggered by the accumulation of permanent damage, i.e., oxidative stress generated by oxidation arising from the association between reactive oxygen species and cell DNA, protein, and lipid components. And as it is observed that the aging mechanism itself is unlinked to oxidative stress; widely frequent chronic age-related illnesses have indeed raised oxidative stress. In herbs, antioxidants can contribute to at least some of their renowned therapeutic effects.

Natural-Derived Analgesic Agents (Natural Products)

Different types of natural ingredients have been used to cure pain problems since the first documented reports, about 7,000 years ago. Examples of those genuine items are opium poppy (*Papaver soniferum*) and willow tree bark (Salix spp.). It was not until the nineteenth century that particular molecules were extracted and believed to obtain the desired results from these chemicals.

The identified origins of such compounds were studied in detail. More analgesic compounds have been removed from natural materials during the last few decades, resulting in new molecular groups and action mechanisms. In drug research attempts, plants or other natural remedies mentioned in historical ethnopharmacological and ethnobotanical literature have been of more recent importance. Such records and studies classify better herbal ingredients, which were traditionally used in pain treatment.

The simple knowledge of the intricate processes of pain transmitting in the nervous system has been a significant factor that has emphasized the significance of finding new compounds to relieve pain. Nociceptive synthesis includes various types of receptors, enzymes, and signaling pathways. Identifying novel groups of compounds through natural sources can contribute to a greater understanding of the pharmacological mechanisms underlying it. With the ability to identify new substances with favorable pharmacological characteristics—i.e., no health risks, no addictive capacity—, natural products also carry tremendous promise for the future of drug development, especially in the treatment of pain conditions and possibly opioid addictions.

Anti-Inflammatory Action of Natural Products

Many inflammatory disorders are being widespread in the world's aging population. The anti-inflammatory medications used clinically suffer from the downside of adverse effects and rising medication costs (in biological drugs). Alternatively, these drugs are natural remedies and natural ingredients which offer great hope in the discovery and production of biologically active lead compounds into medicines for the treatment of inflammatory diseases.

For the prevention of inflammation and other diseases, herbal drugs and phytopharmaceuticals have been used since ancient times. The metabolites listed belong to various chemicals, such as steroids, alkaloids, polyphenolics, and terpenoids, which play a vital role in the anti-inflammatory properties.

Plants Induced Antifungal Agents

A modern *continuum* of human fungal infection is growing because of intensified cancer, AIDS, and patients with an impaired immune system. The increased usage of antifungal agents has also resulted in tolerance to existing medications being developed. New groups of antifungal substances to treat fungal infections continue to be identified. Plants are a rich source of many biologically active secondary metabolites, such as tannins, terpenoids, saponins, flavonoids, alkaloids, and other substances, reported to have antifungal properties in vitro.

Research into natural products and substances extracted from natural resources has also increased in recent years owing to their significance in the discovery of medicines. In plants, which are of considerable value to humans, several compounds have been identified with antifungal action against various strains of fungus. These molecules may be used as a guide to creating better molecules.

Chapter 4. Does the Alkaline Diet Work?

When it comes to diets, you are probably all fed up with hearing about and then trying so many of them, with their promises of incredible results. These "potential" results are usually related to weight loss, and this is something this kind of diet doesn't focus on. The main purpose of the alkaline diet is to improve your health. Of course, if you associate the diet with intense workouts, you will also notice weight loss. And any time the body is functioning at its peak efficiency and health, there will be noticeable effects. Also, unlike other diets, the alkaline diet is best followed permanently, so it's not something to use for a limited period of time. Using the alkaline diet as a life plan may sound a bit discouraging, especially if you have to give up some of your favorite treats. Still, you are gaining a lot of health benefits by following this life plan. It's the smart way to live the rest of your life.

Anti-Aging Effect

There is no known substance that can completely reverse the aging process, but there are several tricks you can use to slow down this process. The alkaline diet is one of these tricks, but it is not a "Fountain of Youth," so you shouldn't expect miracles, as it doesn't add years to your life. It simply helps you feel and look younger and healthier because its effects can be noticed on the skin, nails, and hair. Your skin will regain its radiance and elasticity, your hair will be shinier, and your nails will become stronger.

Increased Vitality and Energy

There is no doubt that the alkaline diet improves your metabolism, and this enhances your vitality. Your digestive system needs the energy to process food and even more to handle acid-forming types of food. Drawing that energy from other body systems puts the whole body into a lethargic state. Balancing the acid/alkaline ratio in your body also increases energy levels because it frees up oxygen for different cells and thereby enhances their functioning.

The alkaline diet stabilizes energy levels throughout the day, avoiding any kind of sugar rush resulting from the consumption of sweeteners, sweets, and sodas. Trying this life plan helps you impose self-discipline because you establish when to eat and what to eat, which will definitely lead to more restful sleep. All of these factors produce a cumulative effect of increased energy and vitality.

Prepares Your Body for Weight Loss

This diet doesn't promise you phenomenal weight loss, but it can set the right conditions for your body to lose weight. The Alkaline Diet can help you reach the natural body weight or BMI (Body Mass Index). It's not designed as a slimming diet, but if you are overweight and have a sluggish metabolism, this diet can speed up your metabolism which can lead to weight loss. You will also eliminate toxins and therefore relieve the fat tissue of the load it's carrying, making it more available to be burned. The alkaline diet also boosts your energy level, which can give you extra motivation to work out and lose weight.

Decreased Bloating and Constipation

Another benefit of this diet, or cure, as some nutritionists like to describe it, is related to your urine and feces. After a short time of living according to the alkaline diet, you will notice soft feces and clear urine, as your body will function properly, and you will become more regular in your bowel movements.

Constipation is something anyone wants to avoid, so if you are experiencing this condition, you should know that the alkaline diet is better than any laxative. It will regulate your bowel movements and, with proper hydration, guarantee a soft stool. The way you eat can also have a serious impact on the work your digestive system does. If you chew your food enough, you make things easy for your digestive system which will be able to properly digest the food, relieving pressure on your stomach and avoiding constipation.

Better Brain Function and Mood

When you feel more energetic and healthier, you also feel better and have a positive attitude. A study conducted by Rudolph Wiley in 1987 proved that acid imbalance can cause all sorts of disorders of psychogenic, psychological, psychosomatic, and stress-related natures. This study demonstrated that an alkaline diet decreased or completely eliminated a symptom's severity for more than 85 participants. Also, this kind of diet consists of plenty of fruits and vegetables, which are rich in vitamins like B6, a very helpful vitamin for your brain function and mood. All the vitamins and minerals which come from the fruits and vegetables of this diet are very helpful for the proper function of your brain and body. Associating this diet with exercise (even if it's not intense) and avoiding as much as possible caffeine, alcohol, and processed food also helps.

A Shield Against Diseases and Allergies

There are plenty of allergies known today which provoke just inflammation in the stomach. Probably the most common allergies are towards peanuts or milk proteins. In such scenarios, the problem-causing food has to be identified, and the system has to be cleansed from it. Then some alkalizing treatments have to be tried on the system. If somebody is experiencing allergies, comprehensive research can discover if the subject is vulnerable to diseases like diabetes, heart disease, or even cancer. There are enough theories which claim that these diseases are favored by an acidic environment, and increased alkalinity can suppress these diseases in an early stage. Also, it is known that veggies and ripe fruits are great sources of antioxidants, which represents the best way to protect you from these kinds of diseases. The bottom line, your immune system is as healthy as your stomach is.

Stronger Bones

If you are experiencing any muscle or bone pain, then the alkaline diet is what you need. It will help you ease your pains and can even prevent or cure osteoporosis, as the diet decreases the bones' acidity with alkalizing minerals. Healthy bones are favored by an alkaline environment, calcium, vitamin D, and weight-bearing exercises.

Enhanced Fertility

Fruits and vegetables with high alkaline levels can seriously improve fertility, for both men and women. The consumption of these foods has amazing effects on the way the reproductive system performs. The body's hormonal system works better in an alkaline environment, leading to better cell function and better fertility. These hormones will enhance the desire for sex, make conception more viable, and promote a healthy pregnancy.

Possible Symptoms or Illnesses Which Can Be Prevented by Using This Type of Diet

There are clearly many benefits to a lifestyle built around an alkaline diet. But the benefits go even further, to impact some of the symptoms, conditions, and illnesses that plague our modern society.

Hypertension, Stroke, and Heart Disease

According to the Centers for Disease Control and Prevention, over 33% of adults have high blood pressure, a condition that increases the risk of heart disease and stroke. While there are a number of risk factors for high blood pressure and heart disease, including inactivity and being overweight, there is a clear and distinct link between what you eat and your risk. The average American diet contains plenty of animal-related products, and it's deficient in vegetables and fruits. This causes an acidosis metabolism and also a low urine pH, but it can also lead to hypertension and even heart disease. With high levels of magnesium and potassium, the alkaline diet contributes to healthy blood pressure. Assuring a high level of minerals through alkalizing foods decreases the risk of heart disease.

Kidney Stones

A recent study estimates that one out of ten people will have kidney stones sooner or later. This statistic is worrying, and if nothing changes in our diet, your risk of being the one increases. The acid environment is the perfect kind of environment for developing kidney stones. Unfortunately, the average diet is high in sodium, animal proteins, and sugar, which are all nutrients that the kidneys have difficulty filtering. Calcium, sodium, oxalate, phosphorus, and uric acid are some of the most common stone promoters. These substances are filtered easily by the kidney of a young person, but as we get older, the kidney doesn't function as it used to.

Eliminating a kidney stone is something extremely painful, but they are avoidable. So, if there is an easy means of prevention, it's crucial to take advantage of it and avoid the extreme discomfort of passing a kidney stone. Therefore, you will need to make sure you consume alkaline food and prevent this from happening. The alkaline cure can be even more useful than consuming beer or wine to prevent and dissolve kidney stones.

Muscle Mass

Aging and a passive lifestyle are the main causes of losing muscle mass. Every person needs a certain number of calories to maintain muscle mass. Losing muscle means that the body will need to consume fewer calories to maintain what it still has, leading to the potential for weight gain if eating habits are not altered. Lost muscle mass also results in less energy to exercise and build back muscles. In other words, muscle loss can eventually lead to more muscle loss, which can definitely affect your mobility, not to mention that you become more vulnerable to fractures and falls. There are two approaches to prevent this from happening. The first one is an increased caloric intake to provide enough energy to work out and increase your muscle mass (protein intake is highly important). Another approach is the alkaline way. A study conducted by the American Journal of Clinical Nutrition discovered that high alkalizing food reduces the acid level and also preserves muscle mass.

As a general rule of thumb, consume vegetables and fruits to get the necessary minerals and vitamins to preserve your muscle mass, mobility, and independence. By doing so, you will be less fragile and less vulnerable to falls or fractures.

Type 2 Diabetes

It is estimated that around 26 million people living in the US have type 2 diabetes and around 10% of adult Americans have this disease, according to the Center for Disease Control and Prevention. Type 2 diabetes is a metabolic disorder in which your blood sugar is higher than normal, and your cells resist the process of balancing blood sugar with the hormone insulin. Luckily, this disease can be prevented if you fully understand its roots and causes.

As studies have shown, the normal high-acid diet is a factor in increasing the risk of this disease. In a study published in *Diabetologia* in 2013, researchers conducted a 14-year cohort study analyzing dietary information collected from a questionnaire from almost 70,000 French women. From the responses, the researchers calculated the PRAL (potential renal acid load) and found a trend correlating a high dietary acid load to an increased risk for type 2 diabetes.

Blood sugar gets high after consuming a large number of carbs, and normally all the excess glucose should be turned into "fuel" and used as energy. Insulin is known as a hormone that turns glucose into energy, and when the body doesn't use insulin or doesn't use it well enough, glucose will remain in the blood, leading to high blood sugar. Coincidence or not, processed foods are rich in carbs, which are considered the main cause of high levels of glucose. They also have a higher acidity, which leads to the conclusion that the acidic food type favors the accumulation of glucose in greater amounts, and at some point, the glucose can't be turned into energy.

Consuming alkaline foods limits the spike in blood sugar because they have a lower concentration of carbs, and the resulting glucose can be easily processed and turned into energy, so it doesn't get stored in the blood. Obviously, this decreases blood sugar and also the risk of having type 2 diabetes.

Chapter 5. Will This Diet Help Me Lose Weight?

Although it wasn't originally made for this purpose, following this diet can help you lose weight. It discourages Western diets that consist mainly of ultra-processed food loaded with sugar, salt, and fat. Instead, it is plant-based, and people that follow it tend to have lower heart disease and obesity rates than those that follow the Western diet.

A 1-year study was done on 65 people. It was found that those who strictly followed the wholefood and low-fat diet lost more weight than those that didn't. After 6 months, those who adhered to this diet had gotten rid of 26 pounds while the others lost 3 pounds.

Furthermore, most of the recommended foods have low-calorie content except for seeds, nuts, oils, and avocados. Therefore, eating large portions of the approved foods won't result in surplus calories. Sadly, most people regain their lost weight as soon as they resume their regular diet.

Does It Help to Reverse Diseases?

The question of whether Dr. Sebi's Diet can reverse diseases is one that still sparks debate today. Alfredo Bowman championed his cause that the diet could provide relief to people with various ailments. Among others, these include diabetes, heart conditions, liver problems, herpes, and kidney issues.

His premise suggested that the foods altered your body's pH and made it more alkaline, thus aiding in fighting disease. Science, however, says otherwise. According to research, foods can alter your urine's alkalinity level, but they do not affect the blood's pH. Still, this does not mean that all is lost. On the contrary, this diet has many health and medical benefits.

Fruits and vegetables improve heart function and strengthen it. It makes the heart capable of combating disease and reduces the risk of heart attacks.

Because the diet is low in fat, it also serves as an excellent way to prevent atherosclerosis and the accumulation of fatty deposits in your blood vessels. Healthy blood vessels allow proper blood flow and minimize strain on your heart.

Your body will also get a healthy balance of macronutrients and vitamins from the listed foods. It fosters an overall improvement in health.

Since this diet is rich in fiber, it can help people suffering from constipation cope with the condition and even reverse it. Seeds, vegetables, fruits, and nuts all play critical roles in easing bowel movements.

Dr. Sebi's Diet has many health benefits, but it comes with several drawbacks. Fortunately, there is a way around them. By consuming plant-based protein sources such as beans and lentils, you can meet the nutritional needs of a well-rounded diet and gain the most benefit. If you suffer from any chronic condition or you are taking certain medications, consult your doctor before transitioning to this diet.

Are There Any Safety Worries About Dr. Sebi Diet?

The Alkaline Diet is a safe diet program. However, it is always smart to look for your healthcare supplier's advice and recommendation before attempting any diet, including the Alkaline Diet. Individuals experiencing acute or interminable kidney disease must not follow this diet except under the physician's guidance and management. Similarly, individuals who had or right now have heart disease, particularly the individuals under medications that affect potassium levels in the body, must not adhere to this diet program without their doctor's approval.

Chapter 6. Tips to Deacidify With the Alkaline Diet

An enormous amount of alkaline diet enthusiasts recommends balanced entire food meals that are more alkaline than acidic. Some individuals allow 80 to 90% of their meals for alkaline foods, while others think it's better to allocate just 60 to 80% for alkaline-framing foods. However, as a general rule, the more you avoid prepared foods, devour more vegetables, leafy greens, fruits, eat fewer lean meats and other protein sources, the easier it is to adhere to an alkaline diet food plan. Also, you may keep the postings of alkaline and acid foods handy, so you can intently screen the foods you are about to place in your system. It presents various ways through which you can transform your usual acidic meals into alkaline ones. In addition, a sample five-day alkaline diet food plan is featured. Finally, four physical activities that can supplement your alkaline diet are examined.

Basic modifications: how to transform foods into an alkaline medium so you won't get overpowered with an abrupt change in diet; there are food modifications you can do. You may use the substitutes underneath to refrain from acid-framing foods and stick to alkaline-shaping ones.

Instead of	Consume This
Canned or glazed natural fruits	Frozen fruits that are liberated from additives
Butter	Cold-squeezed olive oil or clarified butter
Condiment	Fresh flavors and herbs
Coffee	Herbal teas
Creamer	Almond milk
Elating	Agar-agar
Flour	Ground skinless almonds

Peanuts	Chestnuts or almonds
Navy beans	Lentils
Soda	Sparkling water
White potatoes	Sweet potatoes
Sugar	Clover nectar or Stevia
White rice	Basmati or wild rice
Yeast bread	Sprouted grains
Yeast	Lemon juice and baking soda
Red meat	Firm tofu or poultry
Entire eggs	Egg whites

Aside from the above-mentioned replacements, here are different tips by Dr. Sebi on how you could increase your pH level into its alkaline state:

- **Use baking soda:** one of the instant ways to increase the levels of your pH is by drinking a glass of water with some of it. You can add half a teaspoon of baking soda to water at least an hour earlier before any of your meals. You may not know, but they pack most tap water with toxins and are exceptionally acidic. Instead of supporting your body's wellbeing, it can even contrast body activities that help maintain alkalinity, and also reduces some water-related issues.

- **Stay away from handled sugar and grains:** as referenced earlier, they can increase the body's acidity level. You should constrain your utilization of sugar and grain items, such as refined cereals, bread, baked merchandise, and noodles. Instead, devour healthy grains, for example, quinoa, wild rice, millet, and amaranth.

- **Consume fewer dairy items and meat:** if you read the food postings carefully, you see that meat and dairy items are acidic or acid-shaping in the body. Thus, devour healthier protein sources, for example, soy milk, soybeans, soy cheddar, almonds, goat's cheddar, and goat's milk.

- **Make fruits your best diet companions**: again, alluding to the food postings, you see that fruits are an impressive addition to the Alkaline Diet. In particular, citrus fruits, papayas, blueberries, apples, and watermelon are your top decisions. Another decent addition to the diet is raisins. Take note, however, that prunes, cranberries, and blackberries can leave an acidifying impact on the body.

- **Try not to use artificial sugars:** artificial sugars are a guilty party behind the body's wrong pH level. Because of this, instead of utilizing them, attempt to concentrate on natural items, for example, raw sugar, pure maple sugar, nectar, or Stevia sugars. It will also help if you replace diet sodas with herbal teas; these could welcome an enormous difference in your body's level of pH.

- **Play with flavor:** the addition of alkaline flavors can reduce the acid-framing effect of some foods in the body. For instance, you can add paprika to your soups, stocks, or you can hurl nuts with it. Another way is to put bean stew powder on your hot cocoa, it will transform your usual choco drink into a spiced one. When you are having a tuna or turkey salad, you can add parsley for a turn. You can make pan sear dishes, oatmeal, and smoothies tastier and progressively alkaline by blending ground ginger. Finally, you can add curry powder to your usual popcorn.

Dr. Sebi Cell Food

Enhancing Immunity

We are part of nature, developed in helpful interaction with the earth and plants around us. Invulnerable capacities are smothered by non-natural foods and toxins and enhanced when we associate with nature and align activities to natural cycles. The calming sound of the winged animal melody, or the relaxation from watching the sunset, are only two of the ways that the natural world affects the sensory system and enhances the invulnerable capacity.

Rhythms and Cycles

The rotation of the earth and moon create seasonal patterns of light, temperature, and tides. Chrono-immunology aligns the body's master clock to environmental signals and daily variations in a safe capacity. The insusceptible system is progressively active around evening time and is increasingly effective if it can operate while you rest and spotlight all assets on your self-healing.

- **Interruption:** shiftwork, stream lag, and insomnia upset evening time patterns of rejuvenation.
- **Cycles:** sleep and wake cycles are constrained by daylight setting cellular cadenced "timekeepers."
- **Nourishment:** seasonal food gives sustenance aligned with natural patterns and energies.
- **Daylight**: energizes the insusceptible system, lessens inflammation, and synchronizes cycles.

Natural Setting

Our relationship with nature is incredible, so much that observing the shading "green" is relaxing. Survey all the way opens green landscapes, trees, mountains or streams, signals to the body that all is well, assets are bountiful. Being in nature calms the mind, eases back breathing, decreases pulse, relaxes strained eyes, helps oxygen, and encourages insusceptible capacities.

- **Seaside:** sea-air is full of resistance boosting negative particles, which also decreases pressure.

- **Seawater:** rich in magnesium and trace minerals, a dip in the sea is naturally detoxing.

- **Plants:** houseplants channel air, absorb pollutants, and oxygenate during the day.

- **Gardening:** getting near the Earth inoculates you with beneficial soil bacteria.

- **Blossoms**: reduce worry with their fragrance and style, traditionally gifted to speed up healing.

- **Essential oils:** bring the fresh fragrances of outside, inside, thinking back to the senses.

- **Herbs:** create a range of healthful and healing effects, trusted for millennia by Breath, Movement, and Stillness. The lungs are one of the two organs that sit inside both cognizant and subliminal control (the other is the eyes). Breath naturally rises and falls, speeding up and easing back down as required, but you can also control the speed yourself. This dual-control system allows you to take control of your whole physiology by deliberately attending to your breath.

- **Observation**: pay attention to the speed and profundity of your breath.

- **Calming:** slow full breaths, get sustaining oxygen, and evacuate waste carbon dioxide.

- **Development:** gentle development, such as walking, pushes lymph liquid around and out of the body.

- **Ricocheting:** skipping or bouncing back (smaller than expected trampoline) is incredible for siphoning lymph liquid.

- **Resting:** activation of the immune system happens when we are still, mentally, and physically.

- **Fasting:** provides total physiological rest so that the body can concentrate on healing over absorption.

- **Rest:** quality rest is critical to allow the invulnerable system time to work successfully around evening time. By taking a stage back and returning to a slower, increasingly natural, way of life, by default, we settle many of our innovative health issues. Relaxing, tuning in to, and watching natures' beauty, creates ideal conditions for the safe system to flourish. Get outside and bring some outside in, to enhance your resistance naturally.

Feeling Immune

Your safety system is operating every minute of every day of the year to assemble your body, similar to a dynamic work of art. You paint your daily thoughts, feelings, and actions straightforwardly onto the canvas of your beautiful body. Take charge of how you see yourself and your general surroundings.

Habitual Thinking

Personality is the development of various thought patterns with blended needs. Official areas of the brain pick which patterns to comply, and accordingly how to act. Typically, we follow emotionally ingrained patterns from the past, to save mental energy and shield us from harm.

- **Thoughts:** each day, we have about 30,000 thoughts driven by neurological patterns.

- **Negative:** 80% of thoughts are negative, a bias that developed to shield us from harm.

- **Subliminal:** a database of past encounters and emotions that the mind alludes to.

- **Cognizant:** critical speculation based on data and emotions from the past and present.

- **Change:** thinking differently takes mental exertion; this is the reason change feels difficult.

Healthy Habits

Boosting your invulnerability is the natural aftereffect of building healthy habits that help your body to flourish. Avoiding what is bad for health—shoddy nourishment and toxins—and increasing sustenance—alkaline plants and healing herbs—will support your ability to self-heal. The idea is straightforward: it is our pleasure-chasing and habitual mind which disrupts everything. Discovering rewards that don't bargain health, while also being an impetus to keep you on track, is a key bit of the riddle. Trial to perceive what motivates you best, sometimes the basic reward of "ticking off" progress is enough to maintain daily motivation towards a more drawn-out term goal. Resolve to change and reward yourself for the advancement you make, respect the control and exertion you are putting into improving your health.

What to Look Out for When Implementing Dr. Sebi's Diet

For many people hoping to go plant-based, protein is constantly a significant concern. Popular media perpetuated this thought and backed by enormous meat producers that protein is just found in meat. Well, that is not true. Traditional staples, such as nuts, beans, oats, and brown rice, come with an impressive amount of protein. Often, the markets nutrients like calcium as if it's originating from animal-based sources. In all actuality, foods like kale, broccoli, and almonds contain heaps of calcium. Ask yourself: if calcium comes from meat, then where did the animal get it from? It's definitely from the greens they eat. The significant concern for most plant-based diet followers is nutrient B12.

B12, for everyone, is normally present in fortified items, especially cereals and plant-based milk. However, those are not reliable for getting enough of this significant nutrient. The best choice is to take a fluid or sublingual nutrient B12 supplement essentially; to make sure that there are no issues. You can receive a healthy plant-based lifestyle by basing your diet around cooked and crude foods, filled with leafy and bright veggies. These will provide your body with the minerals, nutrients, and cell reinforcements it needs.

Chapter 7. Approved Food Lists

The Sebi's Diet is purely based on a vegan diet, the program focuses on the whole diet form on plants. It emphasizes foods that have been classified as alkaline by Dr. Sebi. It implies that certain plant-based foods are not permitted to be consumed. It is important to be on the authorized food list for all the foods you can eat when following this diet plan. The food list by Dr. Sebi with approved food items is given below:

- **Vegetables:** asparagus, cucumbers, squash, chickpeas, amaranth greens, mushrooms (except shitake), onions, olives, bell peppers, amaranth, okra, avocado, purslane, atones (cherry and plum only), dandelion greens, sea vegetables, (wakame/dulce/arame/hijiki/nori), chayote, tom tomatillo, garbanzo beans, turnip greens, kale, watercress, lettuce (except for iceberg), wild arugula, Mexican squash, zucchini.

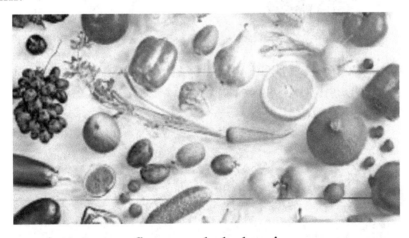

- **Fruits:** apples, pears, figs, seeded cherries, prunes, mango, soft jelly coconuts, cantaloupe, seeded key limes, cactus fruit, papayas, tamarind, plums, seeded grapes, raisins, bananas, peaches, currants, seeded melons, oranges, soursops.

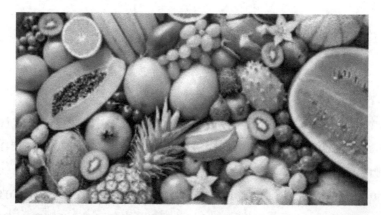

- **Nuts:** raw sesame "tahini" butter, Brazil nuts, hemp seed, raw sesame seeds, walnuts.

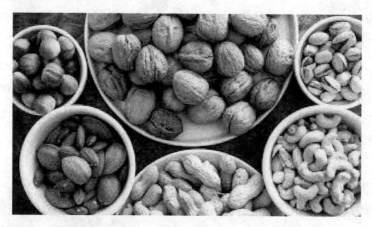

- **Herb:** achiote, basil, onion powder, oregano, bay leaf, sage, habanero cloves, sweet basil, dill, savory, cayenne thyme, tarragon.

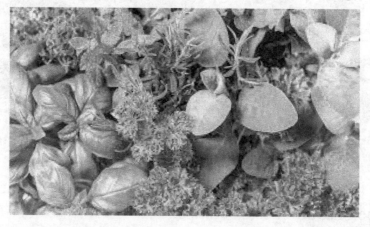

- **Oils:** hemp seed oil, avocado oil, coconut oil (not cooked), grapeseed oil, olive oil (not cooked), sesame oil.

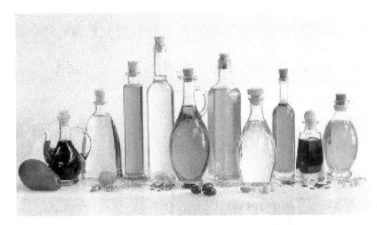

- **Grains:** amaranth, rye, chamomile, burdock, ginger, red raspberry, quinoa, wild rice, herbal teas, fonio, spelt, kamut, tef anise, fennel, elderberry, tila, salt, you may consume the pure sea salt with diet or powdered granulated seaweed.

- **Sweeteners:** alkaline sweeteners. On this food intake, sugar is not permitted, but some alkaline sugar substitutes are allowed. Date glucose (from dried dates) and natural cactus agave syrup can be eaten.

Non-GMO foods:

You should concentrate on foods derived from plants that are untreated or minimally processed. Also, the foods one eats must be non-GMO. Used to prevent pesticides and other additives applied to non-organic foods, it is safer to consume organic food, as much of it as possible. As soon as the foods of preference meet the above requirements, they are likely to eventually allow in the diet of Dr. Sebi.

The Doctor Sebi food list was considered by some dieters to be much restrictive for their taste. Nevertheless, faithful adherents of the diet believe that inside the list there are still enough foods to enable you to have a variety. A traditional Dr. Sebi diet menu might look like veggies pan-seared on either a bed of wild rice, in avocado oil, or a broad green salad with a seasoning of olive oil as well as a hint of agave syrup. Although that can take some time to become used to, the food checklist of Dr. Sebi could be easy to stick to and follow for a healthy diet plan.

Foods You Should Never Eat (and Why)

Below are the main foods items that need to be avoided when following Dr. Sebi's Diet:

- All types of meat, fish and seafood, eggs, wheat, dairy products, fast foods, sugar, seedless fruits, garlic, corn (and products containing corn).

- All types of food that have been processed, GMO foods, any foods that contain artificial food colors and flavors, foods with preservatives, and any type of added vitamins or minerals.

- Soy, poultry, all food items that contain yeast and baking powder.

- Alcohol is strictly prohibited.

As this is a nutritional plan that excludes certain groups of foods, it is essential to use particular nutrients in your diet. Broadly speaking, you might need vitamins including B-12 vitamins, as well as some other vitamins and minerals, like iron, omega-3 fatty acid, and calcium, etc. However, you can get plenty of them from a plant-based diet if you choose them wisely and consume more than one form of plant origin in a single meal; or you may order Dr. Sebi items, which have some herbs and minerals that will offer you vitamins that are lacking in your diet, but visit your physician before trying them. The orders can be placed via Amazon.

List of Herbs Doctor Sebi: Green Food Plus, Sea Moss, Viento and Others

I love how herbal tea consumption has resulted in my general well-being. They help me retain a well-balanced body and have supported one's body to recover itself. Each body is distinct and different herbs will solve the same problem that you might have in various ways, so I recommend that you should do your own research-work and communicating with an herbalist (who understands the African Bio-Mineral Balance) even if you're an herbal medicine specialist or have a name for a disease. Also, the plants I like to use for repair (in no precise order) are the following:

- **Sea moss in conjunction with bladderwrack:** I normally drink it. Use hemp milk, some dates, and cloves to make a special drink from it; 92 out of 102 minerals composing the human body are found in it. I like it wet. It serves to remind me of Milo, kind of thing. I prefer to drink it in the morning and in the evening. Also, I utilize it several times per week to cleanse my face; I simply use spring water to incorporate a dime-sized quantity of powder, end up making it like a paste, and spread this over my face. Around 5 mins or more, I keep it on and rinse. Try regularly our multi-mineral cell which will help you if you don't really like the taste of sea moss.

Dr. Sebi also often spoke favorably for sea moss, it's almost a common diet item that is a part of the daily life for all of us who adopt his diet. He said that it still seems there is uncertainty about which sort of seaweed (species) are called "Irish moss" and how much nutritional value they have today. However, Ireland sea moss, not simple moss may be referred to as a variety of various seaweeds, like (but probably not restricted to) *kappaphycus, Chondrus crispus, alvarezii* (aka *Eucheuma cottonii*) as well as various species inside the genus *Gracilaria*, based on where you live on the planet. *Gigartinales, Chondrus crispus*, and *Cymbopogon alvarezii* refer to the same group, but *Gracilaria* refers to the group of *Gracilariales*.

K. Alvarezii belongs to a group called *Solieriaceae*. In contrast, the Chondrus crispus belongs to *Gigartinaceae's* family, and *Gracilaria* refers to the group of *Gracilariaceae*. Seaweed naming convention utilizes the naming system, a "two-term naming scheme."

Knowing this helps to classify the genus to which a certain species belongs, from their name alone.

- **Dandelion root:** while I have never been a real hardcore coffee addict, I prepare dandelion root tea that tastes quite like coffee whenever I want to feel the flavor. Introduce hemp-milk with date syrup and then you've created a latte for yourself. What's really incredible about it? This is also a liver cleanser. Cleaning up the liver offers you some vitality in return. So, consuming this in the morning is indeed a perfect substitute for coffee, and helps the body to stay in detox mode rather than having all the acid within the body, which coffee drinking can generate.

- **Damiana:** I drink Damiana whenever I feel mentally unbalanced, anxious, or nervous. Even though it is marketed as an herbal remedy, it helps me feel relaxed and not excited. Still, the experience might be unique for others. It's also perfect tea when you're having menstruation. Try Nerves Support in case you are searching for a treatment that can assist you with anxiety and depression.

- **Burdock root:** combo sarsaparilla and burdock root contain up to 102 minerals at low concentrations in the body. To offer me a mineral boost, I want to mix this with other herbs. Because sarsaparilla contains the highest amount of iron and works as a magnet for minerals, I always combine them. (Usually, like linden flower, with a third herb that rounds out the flavor.)

- **Yellow dock:** I introduce this to the tea combos when my skin may feel out of whack, indicating my lymphatic system feels overwhelmed or I have a rash with something I have affected (or touched me). It doesn't always taste fine on its own. I even grind it up and prepare a face mask out of it in a coffee grinder (adding it mainly to sea moss).

- **Blue vervain:** when I feel lacking in magnesium, I drink this. Indications of this are that my brain is overdriving on one problem, and I cannot "wind it off" or I cannot sleep. That relieves anxiety. I typically take out a supplement for Nerve Support in capsule form, since it tastes like a metallic chemical that's not perfect. But I can mix it with damiana or linden as a tea that has a light floral taste. Aside, many people who routinely smoke marijuana are seriously deficient in magnesium.

- **Cascara sagrada:** I recommend drinking it at night, so I'll be ready to go in the morning. I do not recommend drinking it and then moving out for a long period where you'll have to use a toilet in someone else's home. If so, I would suggest covering the smell from some of the bathroom drops, particularly if you consumed some junk in the first place to become constipated.

- **Elderberry:** you can get extremely nauseous when you eat too much elderberry. Also, to get them more appealing, a perfect complement to other herbs.

- **Linden flower:** these are perfect for lung mucus expulsion. Truly calming. When we feel dry throat or a constant cough, it's my time to go. It has a floral taste that is mild. A great compliment to herbal extracts with strong flavors to round out.

- **Black walnut:** normally used to treat parasitic worms, like diphtheria and syphilis, and certain other diseases. It is used for leukemia as well. Some individuals use black walnut mostly as a gargle, apply this as a hair dye into the scalp, or place this on the skin in order to treat wounds.

- **Chickweed:** use this thing for constipation, stomach and bowel issues, and blood disorders along with asthma and other lung-related diseases. It can be used for scurvy and psoriasis as well as scratching, and muscle and joint pain as an enzyme inhibitor. It can be applied for skin conditions including boils, sores, and ulcers.

- **Nettle:** is used for hair growth stimulation. In individuals with diabetes, it helps regulate blood sugar. It decreases gingivitis-related bleeding, treats kidney and helps in recovering urinary tract disorders, and offers water retention. It prevents and handles diarrhea.

- **Mugwort:** it is used to induce digestive juices and bile secretion. It is frequently used to prevent digestive tract diseases and to help with all digestive system issues and is said to have an anti-fungal effect. It has antibacterial, expectorative, and antiasthmatic properties. It can be used in the treatment of a wide range of infectious diseases, like tapeworm, roundworm, and threadworm. Mugwort is thought to be successful. For irregular cycles and other menstrual issues, females take mugwort.

- **Sage:** for digestive issues, including lack of appetite, gas, stomach pain, diarrhea, bloating, and heartburn, sage can be used. It can also be used for minimizing transpiration and saliva increased production, for depression, memory loss, and Alzheimer's disease. It has been used by women for painful menstrual cycles, to fix irregular milk flow during breastfeeding, and to minimize menopausal hot flashes.

- **Sarsaparilla:** for the prevention of gout, gonorrhea, open sores, rheumatoid arthritis, pain in joints, cough, fever, high blood pressure, skin diseases, and indigestion, sarsaparilla is considered effective. It also has the maximum—according to Dr. Sebi—iron content of any herb.

- **Strawberry leaf:** the main use of strawberry leaves is to alleviate gastrointestinal discomfort and joint pain. They include essential minerals, such as iron, an important component of the production of red blood cells, and hemoglobin, which helps to support anemia. It helps in reducing high blood pressure due to its vasodilating effects. It is also advertised as a blood purifier and provides relief from mucus.

- **Bladderwrack:** this is a type of kelp that is used as a therapeutic strategy for obesity and cellulite to activate the thyroid gland. It is rich in iodine and helps to improve metabolism. It also decreases inflammation, improves muscles, enhances circulation, it protects the skin, supports vision, and prevents premature aging. Also, it reduces cancer risk and improves heart health.

In your search for a healthy body, I hope the list provided above will help you. It's a recommendation I want to make to take each herb one at a time and to learn how each one makes you feel personal. Reading books and listening to people is fine but finding it out by yourself helps you with a more intimate view of what is good for you.

The Shopping List of Doctor Sebi's Approved Products

So, you've got Dr. Sebi's Dietary Guidance on board, and you're happy to shop? Few things are fairly easy to locate, but you will have to look a little harder for a few others. You will have to search beyond the model you're used to for conventional food stores, or the big box stores whether you're searching for organic or herbal goods or grains.

Taking the fruits that are approved, such as orange, burro, and baby bananas. You might buy one of these in a normal grocery shop, and you'll notice a bunch more of what you need for this Serbian diet plan if you search a little deeper.

- **Vegetables**: according to Dr. Sebi "Never use the microwave, this will kill all your food."

Amaranth greens, bell peppers, a variety of spinach, dandelion greens, cucumber, avocado, burro banana, asparagus, chayote (Mexican squash), jicama, garbanzo beans (chickpeas), izote (cactus flower/cactus leaf), kale, lettuce (all, but not iceberg), mushrooms (all, but not shitake), mustard greens, olives, onions, okra, squash, nopales (Mexican cactus), poke salad greens, spinach (use sparingly), string beans, tomato (only cherry and plum), tomatillo, turnip greens, zucchini, sea vegetables (dulse/wakame/arame/nori/hijiki).

- **Fruits**: "No canned and seedless fruits." says Dr. Sebi.

Apples, bananas (only the smallest one are allowed or the burro (mid-size original banana), berries complete variety elderberries in any form (but no cranberries), cherries, currants, figs, dates, grapes (seeded), cantaloupe, mango, limes, orange, melons, peaches, pears, plums, prunes, papayas, raisins (seeded), soft jelly coconuts, soursops, sugar apples, cherimoya.

- **Herbal teas:** basil, chamomile, anise, cloves, ginger, lemongrass, red raspberry, sea moss tea, fennel.

- **Spices and seasonings:** mild flavors, bay leaf, cilantro, basil, marjoram, oregano, tarragon, sweet basil, thyme, achiote, cayenne, cumin, coriander, onion powder, sage, dill, salty flavors, pure sea salt, powdered granulated seaweed, kelp/dulce.

- **Sweet flavors:** pure maple syrup—only B grade is recommended—, maple "sugar" (derived from maple syrup), date "sugar" (derived from dates), and pure agave syrup (derived from cactus).

- **Nuts and seeds:** raw almonds, almond butter, raw sesame, raw sesame seeds, "tahini" butter, and walnuts/hazelnut.

It is surprising that people have "allergies to wheat," the reason behind it is not a natural grain; it is produced by science and is a hybrid product, and it is acid-based.

Natural growing grains have a nature of alkaline-based foods; it is therefore recommended that you must use the following products instead of wheat: black rice, amaranth, quinoa, rye, spelt, tef, wild rice, kamut.

Chapter 8. The Benefits That the Alkaline Diet Offers to the Body

One benefit of Dr. Sebi's food regimen is its strong emphasis on plant-based ingredients. The diet promotes eating a wide range of vegetables and fruit, which are excessive in fiber, vitamins, minerals, and plant compounds. Diets wealthy in greens and fruit have been associated with decreased infection and oxidative pressure, similarly to safety in opposition to many sicknesses.

Take a look at 226 people, folks that ate 7 or more servings of veggies and fruit in line with day had a 25% and 31% lower occurrence of most cancers and coronary heart disorder, respectively. Moreover, the majority aren't eating enough produce. In a 2017 file, 9.3% and 12.2% of people met the recommendations for vegetables and fruit, respectively.

Furthermore, Dr. Sebi's Diet promotes ingesting fiber-wealthy entire grains and wholesome fats, which includes nuts, seeds, and plant oils. That food had been linked to a decrease chance of coronary heart disease.

Sooner or later, diets that restrict extraordinarily processed food are associated with a higher common weight-reduction plan fine.

Weight Loss

Despite that Dr. Sebi's alkaline diet is solely not focused on losing weight, strictly following the diet can aid weight loss and prevent obesity. The eating of alkaline food and limiting the intake of acidic foods can make it easy to lose weight. The alkaline diet reduces inflammation and leptin levels that affect fat-burning ability and hunger.

Consuming an alkaline diet, which is an anti-inflammatory food, helps the body achieve primal leptin levels, and helps you feel full of eating a few calories or the amount your body requires.

Reduced Risks of Diseases

The plant-based meals reduced the risk of diabetes, developing metabolic syndrome, improved cardiovascular health, reduced the risk of kidney stones, the risk of coronary heart disease, and memory loss. Dr. Sebi's diet advocates for a meatless diet that is low in calories but high in fiber.

The alkaline diet contains anti-aging effects that decrease inflammation and increase the production of growth hormone.

Lowers Chronic Pain and Inflammation

Chronic acidosis causes headaches, menstrual symptoms, back pains, joint pains, and inflammations. People with chronic pains are treated with daily alkaline supplements for 4 weeks. The alkaline diet is seen to lower chronic pains significantly

Boost Vitamin Absorption

Many people in the world suffer from magnesium deficiency. Magnesium is increasingly required in many body processes and in the functioning of many enzyme systems in the body. Lack of magnesium causes muscle pains, sleep problems, heart complications, and headaches.

Eating an alkaline diet that is rich in magnesium prevents vitamin D deficiency by activating it. Vitamin d is responsible for the overall immune system and functioning of the endocrine.

Protect the Bone Density and Bone Mass

An alkaline diet involves mainly the intake of fruits and vegetables, which are rich in minerals. Eating more mineral-rich foods gives you better protection against sarcopenia, which is muscle wasting and decreased bone strength.

Helps Improve Immune Function and Protect From Cancer

Body cells require minerals to fully oxygenate the body and dispose of waste products from the body. Lack of enough minerals compromise vitamin absorption and helps pathogens and toxins accumulate in the body. This highly weakens the immune system. Alkaline diet sees to it that your body is well packed with minerals, thus boosting your immune system. Moreover, alkalinity in the body helps reduce inflammation and the risk of cancer. Alkaline diet highly benefits chemotherapeutic agents who require high pH to work effectively.

Appetite Control

Eating peas and beans found in the alkaline diet are more fillings than eating animal products like meat. Therefore, eating less alkaline meals can help regulate the amount of food you eat, thus controlling your appetite. This may aid weight loss and overall body health.

Chapter 9. The Disadvantages of the Acid-Base Diet

Although Dr. Sebi's diet promises excellent results, there are some downsides to following the diet. Here are some of these disadvantages:

Lack of Essential Nutrients

Foods listed in Dr. Sebi's diet guide are excellent sources of vital nutrients, carefully selected to help the body stay healthy; however, following this strict alkaline diet may be at risk of a shortage of essential nutrients needed by the human body to function maximally. Although, this diet contains a list of supplements containing proprietary ingredients not listed in the products. This is a call for concern because one cannot determine what nutrients and quantity one should take. This invariably makes it impossible to know if you are meeting the daily requirements of specific nutrients. And some of these nutrients include:

- **Protein deficiency:** this is a critical nutrient needed in the body. It is essential for muscle growth, the brain's health, production of hormones, bones' formation, secretion of enzymes, supports DNA, etc. According to the body's standard requirements to function and develop healthily, people above 19 years of age, either male or female, needs to ingest daily 56 grams and 46 grams.

And although some of the foods listed in this nutritional guide contain protein, they are not significant sources of this all-important nutrient. Some of these Dr. Sebi's approve foods containing protein include: hemp seeds which contain 31.7 grams of protein per 100 grams; 100 grams of walnut would give you 16.8 grams of protein, which is similar to 100 grams of roasted chicken breast. So, for one to be able to meet up the protein requirements of the body, it is advisable to consume a wide variety of foods rich in amino acids (proteins building blocks). But this is not possible because most of the other sources (excellent) of protein are in Dr. Sebi's forbidden food list. This includes meat, lentils, beans, and soy.

To meet up with the body's protein requirements daily, you would have to consume particular, tiring, nearly impossible portions of food when following Dr. Sebi's diet. This will still leave the question of how much quantity and is it enough to meet the nutrient requirements every day.

- **Vitamin B-12 deficiency:** this may happen when a person does not consume enough of this vitamin, which could be another side effect of following Dr. Sebi's diet guide. This vitamin is part of the essential nutrients needed by the body. It functions to maintain the health of the nerves and also the blood cells. It is also critical to the formation of DNA. One of the excellent sources of vitamin B-12 is animal products which are prohibited by Dr. Sebi's diet.

The following symptoms are the result of vitamin B-12 deficiency, a worst-case scenario of possible pernicious anemia, a condition that affects the body by hindering its ability to produce healthy and sufficient red blood cells. Other symptoms are depression, chronic tiredness, and tingling of the feet and hands. Although Dr. Sebi's herbal supplement promises to make up for the missing or inadequate nutrients in the food, because there is no quantitative measure listed on the supplement, one cannot know if one is consuming enough of the required nutrients.

- **Omega-3 fatty acids deficiency:** this nutrient is an essential part of the cell membrane. And it supports the health of the heart, brain, and eyes. It is also a source of energy required by the body for carrying out daily activities, as well as boosting the body's immune system. Although food like walnuts and hemp seeds found in Dr. Sebi's permitted list are plant sources of omega-3 acid, they are not sufficient.

According to research, omega-3 acids are easily absorbed by the body from animal products which are excellent nutrient sources. In order to ensure one is taking a sufficient quantity of omega-3 acids when following Dr. Sebi's diet or any vegan diet for that matter, it is advisable to take an omega-3 supplement daily. This will now lead us to the secondary side effect of following Dr. Sebi's diet.

Insufficient Calories and Negative Eating Habits

Following this diet plan could prove self-defeating because it could lead to negative or poor eating habits. This is as a result of insufficient calories associated with the diet. The diet encourages the use of supplements to balance the missing or inadequate nutrients in the plant-based diet. And supplements do not provide the body with calories. This will lead to under-eating, which could result in several mental, emotional, and physical health issues.

The body needs 1,000 calories to function basically, and this is known as the resting metabolic rate. But when the body engages in physical activities, the body's calories could increase to about 2,000. So, consuming less would lead to slow metabolism, which will eventually lead to low energy. It could also lead to hair loss, constant hunger (which will lead to an unhealthy eating habit), infertility, sleep disorder, irritability, always feeling cold, constipation, and anxiety.

Very Restrictive

Dr. Sebi's nutritional guide is highly restrictive as it forbids so much more food than it permits. It prohibits the consumption of all animal products and some plants, as we have seen earlier. It is so restrictive that it even forbids eating all seedless fruits and even some fruits with seeds (for example cherries).

Lack of Scientific Proof

This is the most important concern with following Dr. Sebi's diet. There is no scientific backing to all the promises of the diet plan. Dr. Sebi claims to change the body's pH—most importantly, the blood pH—through the foods we eat. However, some researches show that while the food we eat could slightly change our urine pH temporarily, it cannot change the pH of the blood and that of the stomach and this is because it needs to maintain a certain level of acidity to carry out digestion. This is one of the reasons some people believe Dr. Sebi to either be a fraud or foolish.

Chapter 10. The Alkaline Diet and Its Relation to Cancer

Dr. Sebi's first step to the cure of cancer was cleansing and detoxifying the body, while the second step is revitalizing it. Sufferers are advised to stop eating foods that are not recommended in Dr. Sebi's food lists if they need to be cured in Dr. Sebi's way.

He recommended detoxification procedures that will remove any form of mucous and toxins in the body. This cleansing and detoxification process involves the employment of Dr. Sebi's herbs that contains strong detoxification agents.

His cleansing and detoxification process is quite holistic because it detoxifies different organs such as the liver, gall bladder, kidney, lymph glands... and many others. Hence, no matter the grade in which breast cancer has developed, the detoxification process will remove all the forms of toxins present.

All the intracellular and intercellular regions of the body will also be detoxified.

Dr. Sebi 21 Days Fasting to Cleanse and Detoxify the Body

To achieve perfect cleansing and detoxification, you must adhere to the following strictly:

- Drink one gallon of water every day.

- Drink tamarind juice each day.

- Constant exercise is needed.

- You must not eat any food other than the ones prescribed in this book.

- When you are done with the detoxification and cleansing process, you are not expected to go back to your wrong eating habits.

- Continue following the alkaline diet even after completing your treatment, as this will help you maintain your health and live longer.

- Ensure you take Irish Sea moss every day.

How to Prepare Irish Moss

- Use warm water to rinse out any attached dirt and debris found in the plant.

- Add 10 cups of clean water to two cupsful of Iris moss.

- Place in a heat source using a large cooking pot and cook for about 25-30 minutes.

- Allow it to become soft and form a paste.

- Add one cupful of water to it again and blend it until smooth.

- Consume it every day.

The herbs Dr. Sebi used for cleansing and detoxification are:

- **Eucalyptus:** cleanses the skin with the use of the steaming process.

- **Rhubarb root:** detoxifies the tone and digestive tract well-being.

- **Dandelion:** detoxifies the kidney and gall bladder.

- **Mullein:** detoxified the lung and activated the lymph circulation in the chest and neck.

- **Elderberry flower:** detoxifies the upper respiratory system and lungs.

- **Chaparral:** detoxifies the lymphatic system and clears heavy metals from the blood and gall bladder.

- **Burdock root:** detoxifies the liver and the lymphatic system.

- **Cascara sagrada:** it helps move stool through the bowels by causing muscle contractions in the intestine.

Preparation of the Herbs and Dosages

- Collect each of the herbs from a reliable source.

- Rinse them thoroughly with clean water.

- Expose them to direct sunlight to make them dry thoroughly.

- Grind each herb separately to powder form.

- Preserve them in a dry and clean container.

- Collect one tsp of each of the above plants and add three cups of alkaline water.

- Boil them for about 5 minutes.

- Remove from the heat source and leave it for a few minutes to get cool.

- Drain before consumption.

- Take one cup of the herb two times daily. It should be taken daily for 21 days.

After you have achieved your detoxification and cleansing, the next step is using herbs needed for the cure of breast cancer.

Let us proceed by describing and introducing the herbs' preparation required for the complete cure.

After 21 days of complete fasting with herbs, water, and juice, Dr. Sebi released the herbs' name that helped cure breast cancer. These herbs are:

- **Sarsaparilla root:** this plant contains a high source of iron that is essential for healing cancer disease.

- **Anamu (Guinea hen weed):** this plant is very effective in fighting cancer cells.

- **Soursop:** this plant is better than chemotherapy, and it fights against cancer. Several types of research had been carried on in this plant to observe its effect on the cancer cell. In one study, they looked at the effect of this plant on leukemia cells, and it was found out that it stopped the growth of these cells. The extract of this plant was also used in a breast cancer cell, and it was observed that the extract was able to diminish the size of the tumor, kill the cancer cells, and made the body immuno-competent.

- **Pao Pereira:** this plant is proven scientifically to kills cancer cells of the breast, ovary, brain, and pancreas. This herb is a great one. It is a tree from the amazon rain forest and is employed as an alternative medication to treat cancer above listed. This plant's extract was applied to a culture; it supports cells' growth, killing the cancer cells. Not only that, but it also caused a total reduction in the size of tumor cells. That means it contains tumor-suppressing activities and can also be utilized for the prevention of cancer disease. This plant attacks only the cancer cells and does not attack other cells as chemotherapy does.

- **Cannabidiol (CBD) oil with tetrahydrocannabinol (THC):** it can also be used to cure cancer. Dr. Sebi used this plant in his village, but in most cases, he does prefer other plants mentioned above.

Chapter 11. Alkaline Water and Cancer

Detox for Cancer Prevention and Cure

To have our cells and tissues regenerated, cleaned, and strengthened, detoxification is the process one must undergo to make this happens, and this is made possible by alkalizing oneself through a raw food diet. Acids and blockages that cause inflammation and block nutrition to our body cells are being removed through this process. Cells are allowed to gain nutritional energy and properly discard waste through cellular respiration due to detoxification, thereby causing the body to rebuild itself.

According to studies conducted, it has been proven that a diet that contains animal protein which is acidic—inflammatory, congestive, and putrefactive —causes cancer. The mucus causes the congestive aspect formed from its putrefactive and abrasive aspects. Vaccinations, toxic chemicals, and hormones fed to these animals or injected into them create tissue toxicity within the body which in turn causes your immune system to be affected by inflammation.

Also, a biochemical imbalance within the body is caused by consuming meat. You begin to experience weakness and dehydration of the body because of the high levels of iron and phosphorus, which eliminates other useful minerals such as magnesium, calcium, and other vital electrolytes needed by the body, thereby making it difficult to trace the presence of cancerous cells that originate from these sources.

The underlining factor here is that over-acidity or inflammation and the build-up of cellular toxicity causes cancer, leading to the loss of cellular energy and function and invariably, the systematic loss of energy and health. The result of this is the overworking of our immune system. The Thymus gland (production site of T-cells) and the bone marrow (production site of B-cell) become hypoactive since it is the tissue responsible for the production of immune cells in a cancer patient.

A Healthy Lymph System Is Needed

Most of the time, 90% of all disease processes begin in your lymphatic system, which is the "sewer system of the body," and a proper understanding of it is a plus. When your system cannot eliminate waste properly because of its congested nature, it then stores the entire waste product in the sewer system, thereby causing a lack of improper elimination of metabolic or cellular wastes, as well as ingested metals and toxic chemicals. Cellular death is bound to occur if these toxins are not eliminated.

First, clean out your lymphatic system so that your immune system can be enhanced for better functionality since the lymph system is a vital part of the immune system. The lymphatic system's channels of secretion are your skin, kidney, and colon; this is worth remembering. You don't remove a septic system that is full or obstructed; you simply clean it out.

Many people don't sweat properly; intestinal bowel walls are impacted and many have lost the proper filtration of their kidneys. All these are simply pointers that the channel of secretion is closed because of its inability to allow waste to be properly eliminated. Since these wastes couldn't get out, they are backed up to the lymphatic system, causing its nodes to enlarge, thus producing all manners of lymphomas, throat cancer, especially having the tonsils removed, non-estrogen types of breast cancer, colon, kidney, liver, and so many problems since this process of always backing up of the waste to the lymph system have been going on for years.

Your cells will begin to strengthen, and the sludge of toxins that kills your cells will be gone by alkalizing and cleansing your fluids and tissues. This is the reason detoxification is important in the elimination of cancer. You will begin to experience vitality, energy, and joy.

There really is no better way to rebuild and clean your body than through detoxification and regeneration of its cells through Dr. Sebi's diet and herbs. There is so much to be accomplished for your life and health if you can just open your heart and take responsibility for your health.

NOTE: Do not have your lymph nodes removed and never compromise your immune system.

Neurological Disorder and Injuries

The highest centers in the body are neurons, and they require the highest energy foods-fruits, acting as an alkaline soil in order to regenerate. Fructose lends its energy effortlessly to your cells since it is a high energy simple sugar. For all neurological issues such as Parkinson's, multiple sclerosis, asthma, and even Bell's palsy, this process is valid.

Through Dr. Sebi's diet and herbs, you can strengthen every cell in your body. To further strengthen the nerve centers, spinal column, and brain tissue, herbal, brain, and nerve formulas of high quality are recommended. Since a great number of our body's neurotransmitters and steroids are created at the adrenal glands, enhancing it is also important.

Considering the thyroid/parathyroid with respect to neurological disorder and injuries. For proper utilization, the parathyroid is needed. Your success is almost guaranteed with Dr. Sebi's diet and good calcium utilization.

With the elimination of over-acidity, pain, cellulitis, deterioration of tissue, obesity, and urinary tract infections, the quality of life of those suffering from nerve damage has been improved greatly or they may experience total recovery at the very best. Don't lose hope that the body cannot regenerate itself again because it can.

The modern food we consume has so much toxin and acid in it and as such makes it difficult for the body to regenerate, due to the high level of mucus, parasite, toxic chemicals, inflammation, and unnecessary hormones. Become alive again by avoiding cooked mucus-forming dairy foods, dead animal flesh, refined sugars, acidic fatty grains whose sole purpose is not to build, but to destroy the body. It is in abstaining from these foods that you begin to experience the miracle of regeneration again.

Chapter 12. Dr. Sebi Diet Recipes

1. Alkaline Blueberry Spelt Pancakes

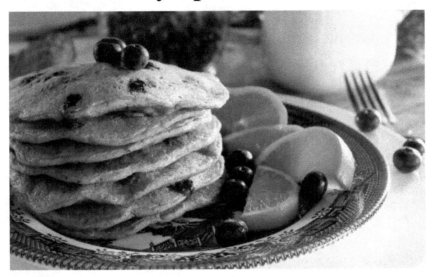

Preparation time: 6 minutes.

Cooking time: 20 minutes.

Servings: 3.

Ingredients:

- 2 cups of spelt flour.
- 1 cup of coconut milk.
- 1/2 cup of alkaline water.
- 2 tbsps. grapeseed oil.
- 1/2 cup of agave.
- hemp seeds
- 1/2 cup of blueberries.
- 1/4 tsp. sea moss.

Preparation:

1. Mix the spelt flour, agave, grape seed oil, hemp seeds, and sea moss in a bowl.

2. To the mixture, add in 1 cup of hemp milk and alkaline water until you get the consistency mixture you like.

3. Crimp the blueberries into the batter.

4. Heat the skillet to moderate heat, then lightly coat it with the grapeseed oil.

5. Pour the batter into the skillet, then let them cook for approximately 5 minutes on every side.

6. Serve and enjoy.

Nutrition:

- Calories: 203.
- Fat: 1.4g.
- Carbs: 41.6g.
- Proteins: 4.8g.

2. Crunchy Quinoa Meal

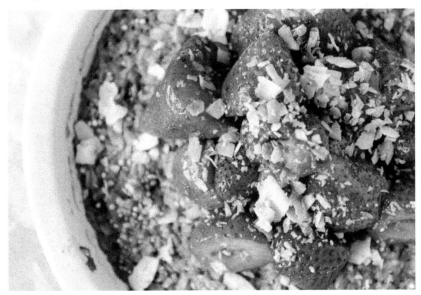

Preparation time: 5 minutes.

Cooking time: 25 minutes.

Servings: 2

Ingredients:

- 3 cups of coconut milk.
- 1 cup of rinsed quinoa.
- 1/8 tsp. ground cinnamon.
- 1 cup of raspberry.

Preparation:

1. In a saucepan, pour milk and bring to a boil over moderate heat.
2. Add the quinoa to the milk and then bring it to a boil once more.
3. Then let it simmer for at least 15 minutes on medium heat until the milk is reduced.
4. Stir in the cinnamon, then mix properly.
5. Cover it. Then cook for 8 minutes until the milk is completely absorbed.

6. Add the raspberry and cook the meal for 30 seconds.

7. Serve and enjoy.

Nutrition:

- Calories: 271.
- Fat: 3.7g.
- Carbs: 54g.
- Proteins: 6.5g.

3. Coconut Pancakes

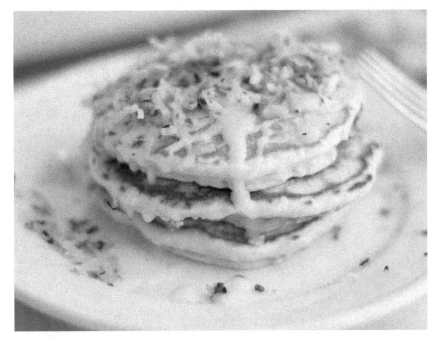

Preparation time: 5 minutes.

Cooking time: 15 minutes.

Servings: 4

Ingredients:

- 1 cup of coconut flour.
- 2 tbsps. arrowroot powder.
- 1 tsp. baking powder.
- 1 cup of coconut milk.
- 3 tbsps. coconut oil.

Preparation:

1. In a medium container, mix in all the dry ingredients.
2. Add the coconut milk and 2 tbsps. of the coconut oil, then mix properly.
3. In a skillet, melt 1 tsp. coconut oil.

4. Pour a ladle of the batter into the skillet, then swirl the pan to spread the batter evenly into a smooth pancake.

5. Cook it for at least 3 minutes on medium heat until it becomes firm.

6. Turn the pancake to the other side, then cook it for another 2 minutes until it turns golden brown.

7. Cook the remaining pancakes in the same process.

8. Serve and enjoy.

Nutrition:

- Calories: 377.
- Fat: 14.9g.
- Carbs: 60.7g.
- Protein: 6.4g.

4. Banana Quinoa Porridge

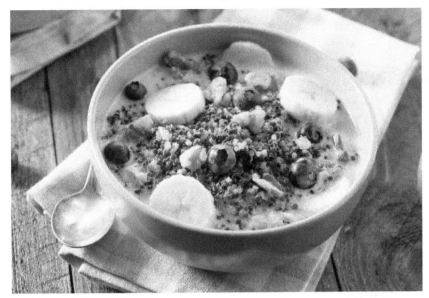

Preparation time: 5 minutes.

Cooking time: 25 minutes.

Servings: 2

Ingredients:

- 2 cups of coconut milk.
- 1 cup of rinsed quinoa.
- 1/8 tsp. ground cinnamon.
- 1 cup of fresh blueberries.

Preparation:

1. In a saucepan, boil the coconut milk over high heat.
2. Add the quinoa to the milk, then bring the mixture to a boil.
3. You then let it simmer for 15 minutes on medium heat until the milk is reduced.
4. Add the cinnamon, then mix it properly in the saucepan.
5. Cover the saucepan and cook for at least 8 minutes until the milk is completely absorbed.

6. Add in the blueberries, then cook for 30 more seconds.

7. Serve and enjoy.

Nutrition:

- Calories: 271.
- Fat: 3.7g.
- Carbs: 54g.
- Protein: 6.5g.

5. Quinoa Porridge

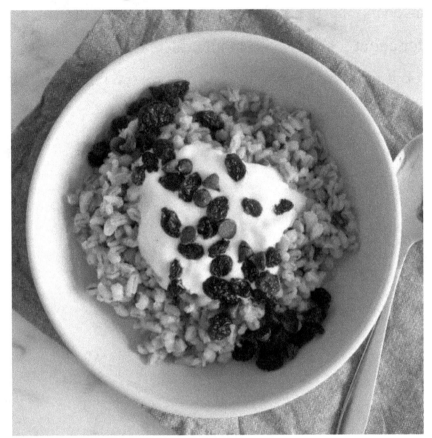

Preparation time: 15 minutes.

Cooking time: 5 minutes.

Servings: 2.

Ingredients:

- 1 cup of divided unsweetened coconut milk.
- 1 small peeled and sliced banana.
- 1/2 cup of barley.
- 3 drops of liquid Stevia.
- 1/4 cup of chopped coconuts.

Preparation:

1. In a bowl, properly mix barley with half of the coconut milk and Stevia.

2. Cover the bowl, then refrigerate for about 6 hours.

3. In a saucepan, mix the barley mixture with coconut milk.

4. Cook for about 5 minutes on moderate heat.

5. Then top it with the chopped coconuts and the banana slices.

6. Serve and enjoy.

Nutrition:

- Calories: 159.
- Fat: 8.4g.
- Carbs: 19.8g.
- Proteins: 4.6g.

6. Zucchini Muffins

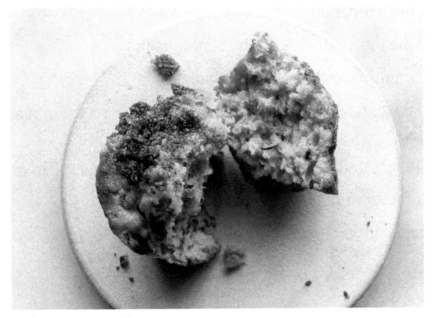

Preparation time: 10 minutes.

Cooking time: 25 minutes.

Servings: 16

Ingredients:

- 1 tbsp. ground flaxseed.
- 3 tbsps. alkaline water.
- 1/4 cup of walnut butter.
- 3 medium over-ripe bananas.
- 2 small grated zucchinis.
- 1/2 cup of coconut milk.
- 1 tsp. vanilla extract.
- 2 cups of coconut flour.
- 1 tbsp. baking powder.
- 1 tsp. cinnamon.
- 1/4 tsp. sea salt.

Preparation:

1. Adjust the temperature of your oven to 375ºF.

2. Grease the muffin tray with the cooking spray.

3. In a bowl, mix the flaxseed with water.

4. In a glass bowl, mash the bananas, then stir in the remaining ingredients.

5. Properly mix and then divide the mixture into the muffin tray.

6. Bake it for 25 minutes.

7. Serve and enjoy.

Nutrition:

- Calories: 127.
- Fat: 6.6g.
- Carbs: 13g.
- Protein: 0.7g.

7. Millet Porridge

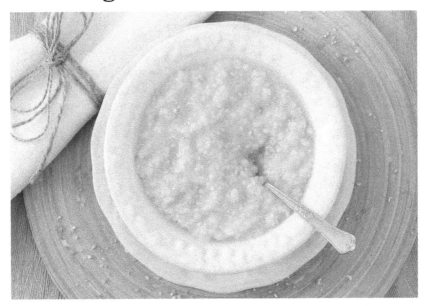

Preparation time: 10 minutes.

Cooking time: 20 minutes.

Servings: 2

Ingredients:

Sea salt.

- 1 tbsp. finely chopped coconuts.
- 1/2 cup of unsweetened coconut milk.
- 1/2 cup of rinsed and drained millet.
- 1–1/2 cu of alkaline water.
- 3 drops of liquid Stevia.

Preparation:

1. Sauté the millet in a non-stick skillet for about 3 minutes.
2. Add salt and water, then stir.
3. Let the meal boil, then reduce the amount of heat.
4. Cook for about 15 minutes, then add the remaining ingredients. Stir.
5. Cook the meal for 4 extra minutes.

6. Serve the meal with a topping of the chopped coconuts.

Nutrition:

- Calories: 219.
- Fat: 4.5g.
- Carbs: 38.2g.
- Protein: 6.4g.

8. Jackfruit Vegetable Fry

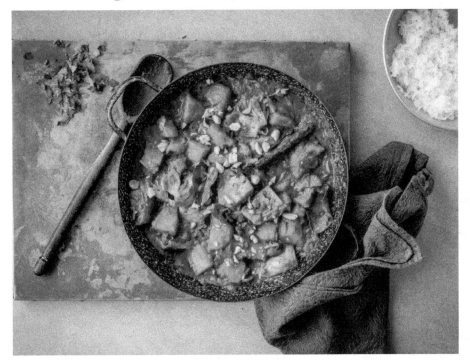

Preparation time: 5 minutes.

Cooking time: 5 minutes.

Servings: 6

Ingredients:

- 2 finely chopped small onions.
- 2 cups of finely chopped cherry tomatoes.
- 1/8 tsp. ground turmeric.
- 1 tbsp. olive oil.
- 2 seeded and chopped red bell peppers.
- 3 cups of seeded and chopped firm jackfruit.
- 1/8 tsp. cayenne pepper.
- 2 tbsps. chopped fresh basil leaves.
- Salt.

Preparation:

1. In a greased skillet, sauté the onions and bell peppers for about 5 minutes.

2. Add the tomatoes, then stir.

3. Cook for 2 minutes.

4. Then add the jackfruit, cayenne pepper, salt, and turmeric.

5. Cook for about 8 minutes.

6. Garnish the meal with basil leaves.

7. Serve warm and enjoy.

Nutrition:

- Calories: 236.
- Fat: 1.8g.
- Carbs: 48.3g.
- Protein: 7g.

9. Zucchini Pancakes

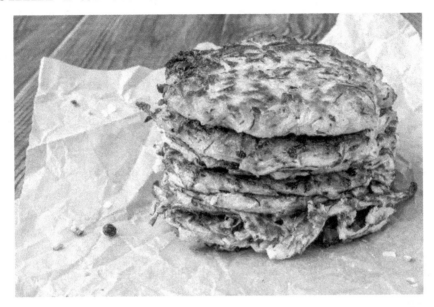

Preparation time: 15 minutes.

Cooking time: 8 minutes.

Servings: 8.

Ingredients:

- 12 tbsps. alkaline water.
- 6 large grated zucchinis.
- Sea salt.
- 4 tbsps. ground flax seeds.
- 2 tsp. olive oil.
- 2 finely chopped jalapeño peppers.
- black pepper
- 1/2 cup of finely chopped scallions.

Preparation:

1. In a bowl, mix water, scallion, and the flax seeds; then set it aside.
2. Pour oil into a large non-stick skillet, then heat it on medium heat.
3. Add the black pepper, salt, and zucchini.

4. Cook for 3 minutes, then transfer the zucchini into a large bowl.

5. Add the flaxseed and the scallion mixture, then properly mix it.

6. Preheat a griddle, then grease it lightly with the cooking spray.

7. Pour 1/4 of the zucchini mixture into a griddle, then cook for 3 minutes.

8. Flip the side carefully, then cook for 2 more minutes.

9. Repeat the procedure with the remaining mixture in batches.

10. Serve and enjoy.

Nutrition:

- Calories: 71.
- Fat: 2.8g.
- Carbs: 9.8g.
- Protein: 3.7g.

10. Squash Hash

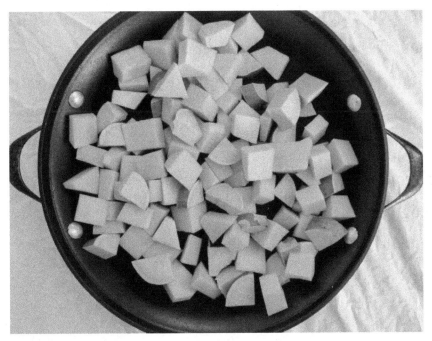

Preparation time: 2 minutes.

Cooking time: 10 minutes.

Servings: 2.

Ingredients:

- 1 tsp. onion powder.
- 1/2 cup of finely chopped onion.
- 2 cups of spaghetti squash.
- 1/2 tsp. sea salt.

Preparation:

1. Using paper towels, squeeze extra moisture from spaghetti squash.
2. Place the squash into a bowl, then add the salt, onion, and the onion powder.
3. Stir properly to mix them.
4. Spray a non-stick cooking skillet with cooking spray, then place it over moderate heat.

5. Add the spaghetti squash to the pan.

6. Cook the squash for about 5 minutes.

7. Flip the hash browns using a spatula.

8. Cook for an extra 5 minutes until the desired crispness is reached.

9. Serve and enjoy.

Nutrition:

- Calories: 44.

- Fat: 0.6g.

- Carbs: 9.7g.

- Protein: 0.9g.

11. Hemp Seed Porridge

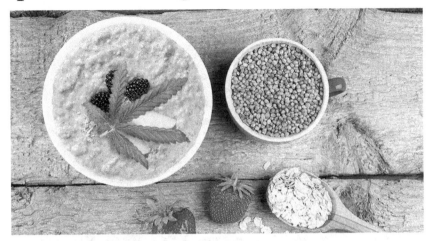

Preparation time: 5 minutes.

Cooking time: 5 minutes.

Servings: 6.

Ingredients:

- 3 cups of cooked hemp seed.
- 1 packet Stevia.
- 1 cup of coconut milk.

Preparation:

1. In a saucepan, mix the hemp seed and the coconut milk over moderate heat for about 5 minutes as you stir it constantly.

2. Remove the pan from the heat, then add the Stevia. Stir.

3. Serve in 6 bowls and enjoy.

Nutrition:

- Calories: 236.
- Fat: 1.8g.
- Carbs: 48.3g.
- Protein: 7g.

12. Veggie Medley

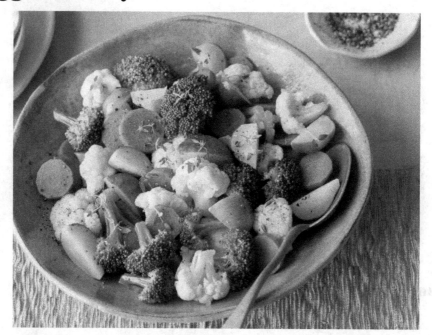

Preparation time: 5 minutes.

Cooking time: 10 minutes.

Servings: 2.

Ingredients:

- 1 seeded and sliced bell pepper.
- 1/2 cup of lime juice.
- 2 tbsps. fresh cilantro.
- 1/2 tsp. cumin.
- 1 tsp. sea salt.
- 1 chopped jalapeño.
- 1/2 cup of sliced zucchini.
- 1 cup of halved cherry tomatoes.
- 1/2 cup of sliced mushrooms.
- 1 cup of cooked broccoli florets.
- 1 chopped sweet onion.

Preparation:

1. Spray a non-stick pan with cooking spray, then place it over moderate heat.

2. Add the broccoli, tomatoes, bell pepper, onion, zucchini, jalapeno, and mushrooms.

3. Cook for about 7 minutes as you stir it occasionally.

4. Add in the cilantro, cumin, and salt, then stir.

5. Cook for an extra 3 minutes while stirring.

6. Remove pan from heat, then add the lime juice.

7. Serve and enjoy.

Nutrition:

1. Calories: 86.

2. Fat: 0.07g.

3. Carbs: 17.4g.

4. Protein: 4.1g.

13. Alkaline Blueberry Breakfast Cake

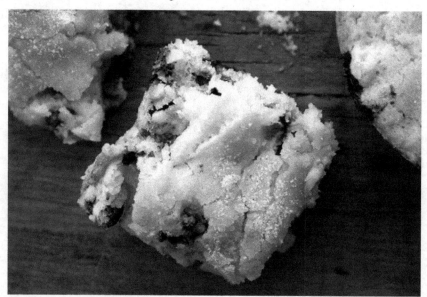

Preparation time: 15 minutes.

Cooking time: 7 hours.

Servings: 6.

Ingredients:

- 1 tbsp. grapeseed oil.
- 3/4 cup of spelt flour.
- 3/4 cup of Teff flour.
- 1/4 tsp. sea salt.
- 1 cup of coconut milk.
- 1/3 cup of agave.
- 1/2 cup of fresh blueberries.

Preparation:

1. Grease a cake pan with grapeseed oil and line with parchment paper. Set aside. Make sure that the cake pan will fit inside the instant pot.

2. In a bowl, mix the spelt and teff flour. Add the salt and stir to combine everything.

3. In another bowl, combine the milk and agave.

4. Stir the wet ingredients to the dry ingredients and fold until well-combined or until the lumps are formed.

5. Add in the blueberries last.

6. Pour the batter into the prepared cake pan.

7. Place in the instant pot and close the lid. Make sure that the vent is not set to the sealing position.

8. Adjust the cooking time to 7 hours.

9. Serve and enjoy.

Nutrition:

- Calories: 293.
- Protein: 7.4g.
- Carbs: 39.8g.
- Sugar: 7.6g.
- Fat: 13g.

14. Zucchini Bacon

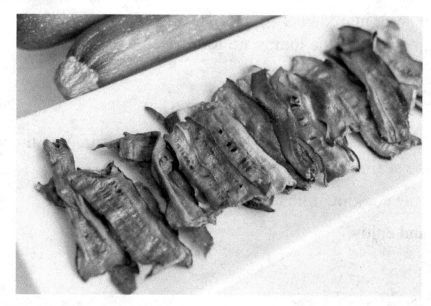

Preparation time: 10 minutes.

Cooking time: 6 minutes.

Servings: 4.

Ingredients:

- 3 zucchinis, sliced thinly lengthwise or into large strips.
- 1/4 cup of date sugar.
- 1/4 cup of spring water.
- 1 tbsp. sea salt.
- 1 tbsp. onion powder.
- 1/2 tsp. cayenne pepper powder.
- 1/2 tsp. ground ginger.
- 1 tbsp. liquid smoke.
- Grapeseed oil for frying.

Preparation:

1. Place all ingredients except for the grapeseed oil in a bowl.
2. Allow the zucchini strips to marinate for at least 2 hours in the fridge.

3. On the instant pot, press the sauté button and heat the oil until it slightly smokes.

4. Fry the marinated zucchini strips for 3 minutes on each side until crispy.

5. Serve and enjoy.

Nutrition:

- Calories: 36.
- Protein: 0.64g.
- Carbs: 8.7g.
- Sugar: 6.5g.
- Fat: 0.09g.

15. Alkaline Spelt Bread

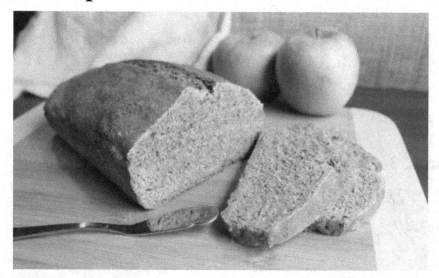

Preparation time: 15 minutes.

Cooking time: 6 hours.

Servings: 8.

Ingredients:

- 4–1/2 cups of spelt flour.
- 2 teaspoons sea salt.
- 2 cups of spring water.
- 1/4 cup of agave.
- Grapeseed oil for brushing the bread.
- A dash of sesame seeds.

Preparation:

1. Use the hook attachment of the mixer to mix the ingredients.
2. In a bowl, mix the spelt flour and salt. Place in a mixer and mix for 10 seconds.
3. Add in the water and agave. Mix for 10 minutes until the dough is formed.
4. Coat the dough with grapeseed oil and place in a clean bowl. Allow resting for at least 1 hour.

5. Line the bottom of the instant pot with parchment paper.

6. Sprinkle the dough with sesame seeds and place inside the instant pot.

7. Close the lid but do not set the vent to the sealing position.

8. Press the slow cook button and adjust the cooking time to 6 hours.

9. Serve and enjoy.

Nutrition:

- Calories: 331.
- Protein: 14.3g.
- Carbs: 68.7g.
- Sugar: 6.7g.
- Fat: 2.4g.

16. Alkaline Crustless Quiche

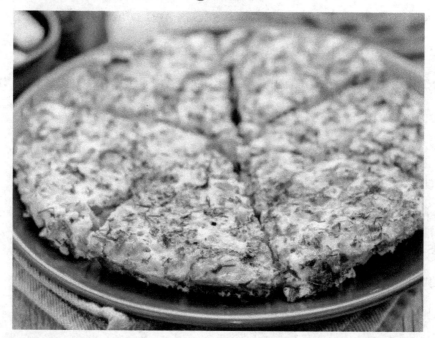

Preparation time: 15 minutes.

Cooking time: 4 hours.

Servings: 4.

Ingredients:

- 1 cup of garbanzos bean flour.
- 3/4 cup of fresh coconut milk.
- 1 tbsp. sea salt.
- 1 tbsp. oregano.
- 1/4 tsp. cayenne pepper.
- 2 cups of mushrooms, sliced.
- 1 cup of kale, chopped.
- 1/2 cup of white onions, chopped.
- 1/2 cup of yellow peppers, seeded and chopped.

Preparation:

1. Place the garbanzos bean flour, coconut milk, salt, oregano, and cayenne pepper. Mix until a smooth batter is formed.

2. Stir in the rest of the ingredients.

3. Place a parchment paper in the bottom of the instant pot and pour over the mixture.

4. Close the lid but do not set the vent to the sealing position.

5. Press the slow cook button and adjust the cooking time to 4 hours.

6. Serve and enjoy.

Nutrition:

- Calories: 328.
- Protein: 12.1g.
- Carbs: 40g.
- Sugar: 7.3g.
- Fat: 14.9g.

17. Dr. Sebi's Home Fries

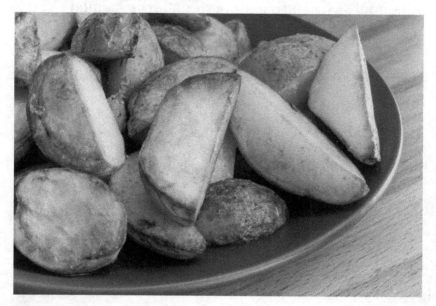

Preparation time: 15 minutes.

Cooking time: 6 minutes.

Servings: 6.

Ingredients:

- 3 green bananas, peeled and chopped.
- 1/4 cup of onion, diced.
- 1/4 cup of green pepper, seeded and diced.
- 1 plum tomato, diced.
- 1 tsp. sea salt.
- 1 tsp. oregano.
- 1/2 tsp. cayenne powder.
- Grapeseed oil for frying.

Preparation:

1. Place all ingredients except for the grapeseed oil in a bowl. Mix until well-combined.

2. Press the sauté button on the instant pot and heat the oil.

3. Get a tablespoon of the mixture and place it in the instant pot. Flatten to form a small pancake.

4. Cook for 3 minutes on all sides.

5. Do the same thing to the rest of the mixture.

6. Serve and enjoy.

Nutrition:

- Calories: 77.
- Protein: 0.66g.
- Carbs: 13.4g.
- Sugar: 7.8 g.
- Fat: 3g.

18. Alkaline Blueberry and Strawberry Muffins

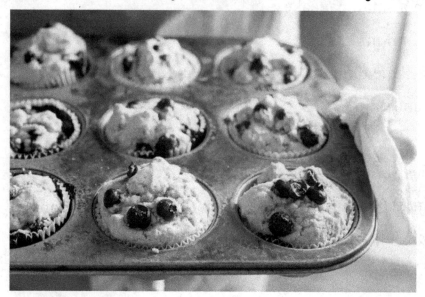

Preparation time: 15 minutes.

Cooking time: 5 hours.

Servings: 6

Ingredients:

- 3/4 cup of quinoa flour.
- 3/4 cup of Teff flour.
- 1/2 tsp. salt.
- 1/3 cup of agave.
- 1 cup of fresh coconut milk.
- 1/4 cup of strawberries, chopped.
- 1/4 cup of blueberries.

Preparation:

1. Place the quinoa flour, teff flour, and salt in a bowl.

2. In another bowl, combine the agave and coconut milk. Slowly pour the wet ingredients into the dry ingredients.

3. Mix until well-combined.

4. Stir in the berries and mix until well-combined.

5. Pour the batter into muffin pans.

6. Place the muffin pans with the batter in the instant pot.

7. Close the lid but do not set the vent to the sealing position.

8. Press the slow cook button and adjust the cooking time to 4 to 5 hours.

9. Serve and enjoy.

Nutrition:

- Calories: 271.
- Protein: 7.2g.
- Carbs: 36.6g.
- Sugar: 4.3g.
- Fat: 11.5 g.

19. Teff Breakfast Porridge

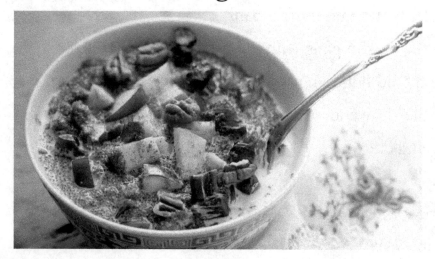

Preparation time: 15 minutes.

Cooking time: 10 minutes.

Servings: 4.

Ingredients:

- 1/2 cup of Teff grain.
- 2 cups of spring water.
- A pinch of sea salt.
- 1/2 cup of agave.
- 1/4 cup of fresh blueberries.

Preparation:

1. Place the teff grain and spring water in the instant pot. Stir in the sea salt.
2. Close the lid and set the vent to the sealing position.
3. Press the multigrain button and adjust the cooking time to 10 minutes. Cook on high.
4. Once the timer sets off, do the natural pressure release.
5. Place the porridge in bowls and drizzle with agave. Top with blueberries.

6. Serve and enjoy.

Nutrition:

- Calories: 105.
- Protein: 3.3g.
- Carbs: 21.8g.
- Sugar: 3.8g.
- Fat: 0.6 g.

20. Alkaline Sausage Links

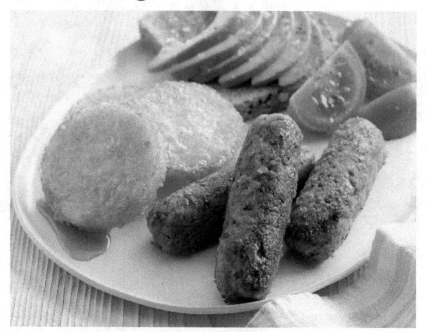

Preparation time: 15 minutes.

Cooking time: 6 minutes.

Servings: 6.

Ingredients:

- 2 cups of garbanzos beans flour.
- 1 cup of chopped mushrooms.
- 1/2 cup of chopped onions.
- 1 tomato, chopped.
- 1 tsp. oregano.
- 1 tsp. sea salt.
- 1 tsp. ground sage.
- 1 tsp. dill, chopped.
- 1/2 tsp. cayenne pepper powder.
- Grapeseed oil for frying.

Preparation:

1. Place all ingredients in a bowl except for the grapeseed oil.

2. Use your hands and mix all ingredients until well-combined.

3. Create small logs of sausages and place them inside the fridge to set for at least 30 minutes.

4. Pour oil into the instant pot and press the sauté button until the oil is hot.

5. Place the sausage links carefully and cook on all sides for 3 minutes.

6. Serve and enjoy.

Nutrition:

- Calories: 266.
- Protein: 14.6g.
- Carbs: 44.9g.
- Sugar: 8.6g.
- Fat: 4.2g.

21. Breakfast Blackberry Bars

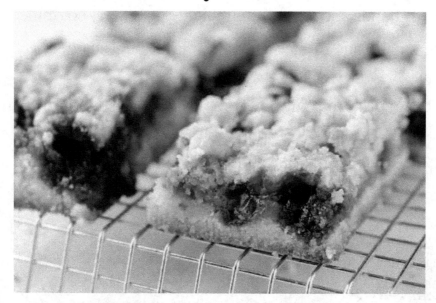

Preparation time: 15 minutes.

Cooking time: 6 hours.

Servings: 8.

Ingredients:

- 4 baby bananas, ripe.
- 1/2 cup of grapeseed oil.
- 1/4 cup of agave nectar.
- 2 cups of quinoa flakes.
- 1 cup of spelt flour.
- 1/4 tsp. sea salt.
- 1/2 cup of blackberry fruits.

Preparation:

1. Place the bananas, grapeseed oil, and agave. Stir and mash the banana until combined.

2. Add the quinoa flakes and spelt flour into the bananas. Add the salt and blackberry last.

3. Place the mixture in a parchment-lined bottom of the instant pot.

4. Close the lid but do not set the vent to the sealing position.

5. Press the slow cook button and adjust the cooking time to 5 to 6 hours.

6. Once cooked, allow cooling before removing and slicing into bars.

7. Serve and enjoy.

Nutrition:

- Calories: 433.
- Protein: 9.9g.
- Carbs: 57.3g.
- Sugar: 10.5g.
- Fat: 19.7g.

22. Butternut Squash Hash Browns

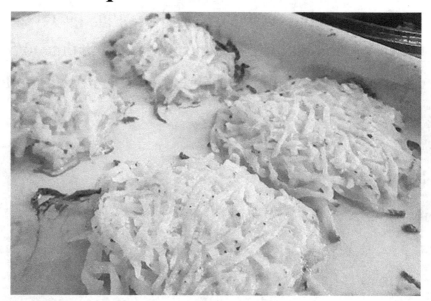

Preparation time: 15 minutes.

Cooking time: 6 minutes.

Servings: 3.

Ingredients:

- 1/2 cup of butternut squash.

- 1/2 cup of diced onion.

- A dash of sea salt.

- A dash of cayenne pepper powder.

- Grapeseed oil for brushing the instant pot.

Preparation:

1. Shred the butternut squash and place in a bowl.

2. Add the onion, salt, and cayenne pepper.

3. Mix until well-combined.

4. Create small patties using the mixture.

5. Pour grapeseed oil into the instant pot and press the sauté button.

6. Place the hash brown in the instant pot and cook for 3 minutes on all sides.

7. Serve and enjoy.

Nutrition:

- Calories: 64.
- Protein: 0.7g.
- Carbs: 5.9g.
- Sugar: 2.1g.
- Fat: 4.6 g.

23. Blueberry Spelt Flat Cakes

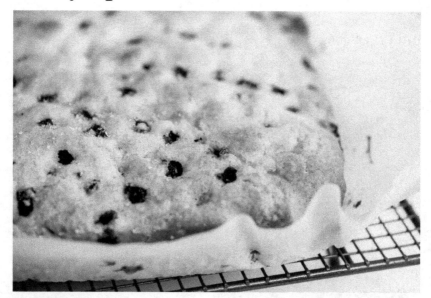

Preparation time: 15 minutes

Cooking time: 4 hours

Servings: 4

Ingredients:

- 2 cups of spelt flour.
- 1/4 tsp. sea salt.
- 1/4 cup of hemp seeds.
- 1 cup of fresh coconut milk.
- 1/2 cup of spring water.
- 2 tbsps. grapeseed oil.
- 1/2 cup of agave.
- 1/2 cup of blueberries.

Preparation:

1. In a bowl, mix the spelt flour, sea salt, and hemp seeds.

2. Pour in the coconut milk, water, grapeseed oil, and agave.

3. Stir until well-combined. Pour in the blueberries.

4. Line the instant pot with parchment paper.

5. Pour the batter into the instant pot.

6. Close the lid but do not set the vent to the sealing position.

7. Press the slow cook button and adjust the cooking time to 4 hours.

8. Serve and enjoy.

Nutrition:

- Calories: 574.
- Protein: 16.1g.
- Carbs: 74.8g.
- Sugar: 14.8g.
- Fat: 27.8g.

24. Breakfast Quinoa Cereal

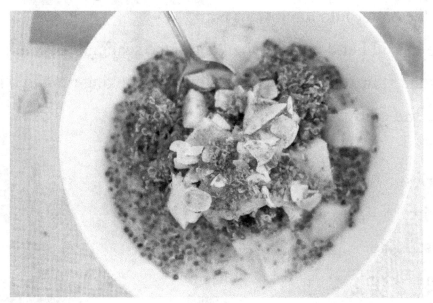

Preparation time: 15 minutes.

Cooking time: 15 minutes.

Servings: 2.

Ingredients:

- 1 cup of quinoa.
- 2 cups of spring water.
- A dash of cayenne pepper.
- A dash of sea salt.
- A dash of oregano.

Preparation:

1. Place the quinoa and spring water in the instant pot. Give a good stir.
2. Close the lid and set the vent to the sealing position.
3. Press the multigrain button and adjust the cooking time to 15 minutes.
4. Do natural pressure release.
5. Once the lid is open, ladle the porridge in bowls and top with cayenne pepper, salt, and oregano.

6. Serve and enjoy.

Nutrition:

- Calories: 322.
- Protein: 12.45g.
- Carbs: 56.7g.
- Sugar: 1.2g.
- Fat: 5.2g.

25. Sweet Date Quinoa Porridge

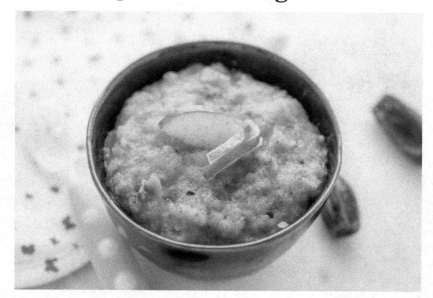

Preparation time: 5 minutes.

Cooking time: 20 minutes.

Servings: 2.

Ingredients:

- 1 cup of rolled quinoa flakes.
- 2 cups of water.
- 1/8 tsp. sea salt.
- 1 cup of fresh dates, pitted and chopped.

Preparation:

1. Place all ingredients in the instant pot. Give a good stir.
2. Close the lid and set the vent to the sealing position.
3. Press the multigrain button and adjust the cooking time to 15 minutes.
4. Do natural pressure release.
5. Serve and enjoy.

Nutrition:

- Calories: 520.

- Protein: 13.8g.
- Carbs: 109.7g.
- Sugar: 46.5g.
- Fat: 5.5g.

26. Turnip Green Soup

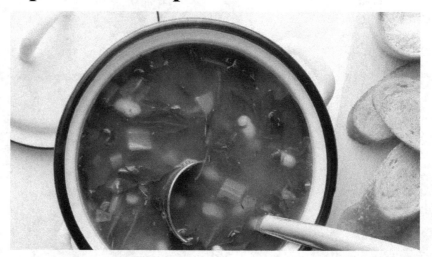

Preparation time: 5 minutes.

Cooking time: 22 minutes.

Servings: 2.

Ingredients:

- 2 tbsps. coconut oil.
- 1 large chopped onion.
- 3 minced chive cloves.
- 2-in piece peeled and minced ginger.
- 3 cups of bone broth.
- 1 medium cubed white turnip.
- 1 large chopped head radish.
- 1 bunch chopped kale.
- 1 Seville orange, 1/2 zested and juice reserved.
- 1/2 tsp. sea salt.
- 1 bunch of cilantro.

Preparation:

1. In a skillet, add oil, then heat it. Add in the onions as you stir. Sauté for about 7 minutes, then add chive and ginger. Cook for about 1 minute.

2. Add in the turnip, broth, and radish, then stir. Bring the soup to a boil, then reduce the heat to allow it to simmer. Cook for an extra 15 minutes, then turn off the heat.

3. Pour in the remaining ingredients, then using a handheld blender, pour the mixture. Garnish with cilantro.

4. Serve warm and enjoy.

Nutrition:

- Calories: 249.
- Fat: 11.9g.
- Carbs: 1.8g.
- Protein: 35g.

27. Lentil Kale Soup

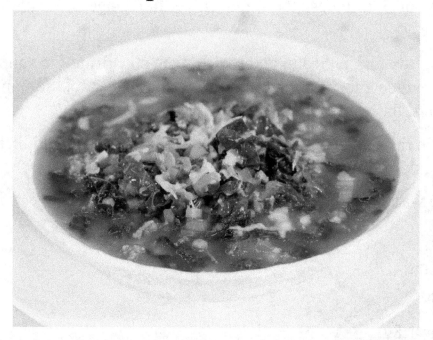

Preparation time: 5 minutes.

Cooking time: 15 minutes.

Servings: 4.

Ingredients:

- 1/2 onion.
- 2 zucchinis.
- 1 rib celery.
- 1 chive stalk.
- 1 cup of diced tomatoes.
- 1 tsp. dried vegetable broth powder.
- 1 tsp. sazon seasoning.
- 1 cup of red lentils.
- 1 tbsp. Seville orange juice.
- 3 cups of alkaline water.
- 1 bunch kale.

Preparation:

1. In a greased pan, pour in all the vegetables. Sauté for about 5 minutes, then add the tomatoes, broth, and sazon seasoning.

2. Mix properly, then stir in the red lentils with water. Cook until the lentils become soft and tender.

3. Add the kale, then cook for about 2 minutes.

4. Serve warm with the Seville orange juice and enjoy.

Nutrition:

- Calories: 301.
- Fat: 12.2g.
- Carbs: 15g.
- Protein: 28.8g.

28. Tangy Lentil Soup

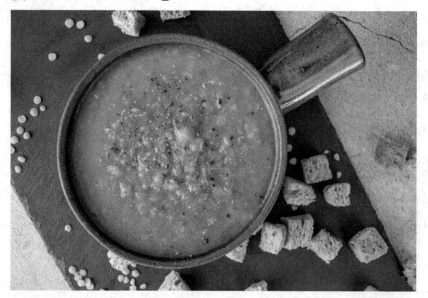

Preparation time: 5 minutes.

Cooking time: 15 minutes.

Servings: 4.

Ingredients:

- 2 cups of picked over and rinsed red lentils.
- 1 chopped serrano chili pepper.
- 1 large chopped and roughly tomato.
- 1–1/2 inch peeled and grated piece of ginger.
- 3 finely chopped chive cloves.
- 1/4 tsp. ground turmeric.
- Sea salt.

Topping:

- 1/4 cup of coconut yogurt.

Preparation:

1. In a pot, add the lentils with enough water to cover the lentils. Boil the lentils, then reduce the heat.

2. Cook within 10 minutes on low heat to simmer. Add the remaining ingredients, then stir.

3. Cook until lentils become soft and adequately mixed. Garnish a dollop of coconut yogurt.

4. Serve and enjoy.

Nutrition:

- Calories: 248.
- Fat: 2.4g.
- Carbs: 12.2g.
- Protein: 44.3g.

29. Vegetable Casserole

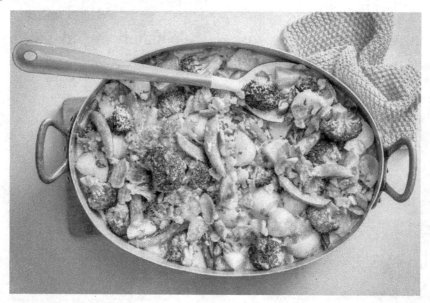

Preparation time: 5 minutes.

Cooking time: 1 hour and 30 minutes.

Servings: 6

Ingredients:

- 2 large peeled and sliced eggplants.
- Sea salt.
- 2 large diced cucumbers.
- 2 small diced green peppers.
- 1 small diced red pepper.
- 1 small diced yellow pepper.
- 1/4 lb. sliced green beans.
- 1/2 cup of olive oil.
- 2 large chopped sweet onions.
- 3 crushed chive cloves.
- 2 cubed yellow squash.
- 20 halved cherry tomatoes.

- 1/2 tsp. sea salt.
- 1/4 tsp. fresh ground pepper.
- 1/4 cup of alkaline water.
- 1 cup of fresh seasoned breadcrumbs.

Preparation:

1. Set the temperature to 350° F of your oven. Mix the eggplant with salt, then keep it aside.

2. Heat a greased skillet, then sautés the eggplant until it is evenly browned.

3. Transfer the eggplant to a separate plate. Sauté the onions in the same pan until it becomes soft.

4. Add the chive, then stir. Cook within a minute, then turn off the heat.

5. Layer a greased casserole dish with eggplants, yellow squash, cucumbers, peppers, and green beans. Add the onion mixture, tomatoes, pepper, and salt.

6. Sprinkle the seasoned breadcrumbs as toppings. Bake for an hour and 30 minutes.

7. Serve and enjoy.

Nutrition:

- Calories: 372.
- Fat: 11.1g.
- Carbs: 0.9g.
- Protein: 63.5g.

30. Mushroom Leek Soup

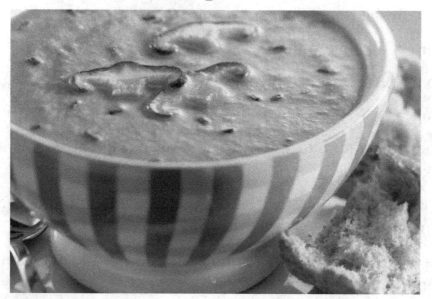

Preparation time: 5 minutes.

Cooking time: 8 minutes.

Servings: 4.

Ingredients:

- 3 tbsps. divided vegetable oil. 2–
- 3/4 cups of finely chopped leeks.3
- finely minced chive stalks.
- 7 cups of cleaned and sliced assorted mushrooms.
- 5 tbsps. coconut flour.
- 3/4 tsp. sea salt.
- 1/2 tsp. ground black pepper.
- 1 tbsp. finely minced fresh dill.
- 3 cups of vegetable broth.
- 2/3 cup of coconut cream.
- 1/2 cup of coconut milk.
- 1–1/2 tbsps. sherry vinegar.

Preparation:

1. Preheat oil in a Dutch oven, then sauté the leeks and chive until they become soft. Add in the mushrooms, then stir. Sauté for about 10 minutes.

2. Add pepper, dill, flour, and salt. Mix properly, then cook for about 2 minutes. Pour in the broth, then cook to boil.

3. Reduce the heat in the oven, then add the remaining ingredients.

4. Serve warm with coconut flour bread and enjoy.

Nutrition:

- Calories: 127.
- Fat: 3.5g.
- Carbs: 3.6g.
- Protein: 21.5g.

31. Red Lentil Squash Soup

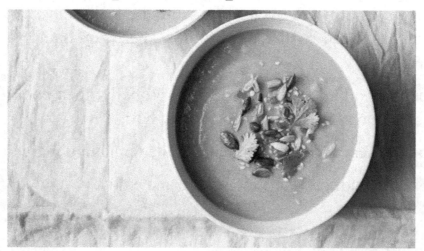

Preparation time: 5 minutes.

Cooking time: 4 minutes.

Servings: 4.

Ingredients:

- 1 chopped yellow onion.
- 2 tbsps. olive oil.
- 1 large diced butternut squash.
- 1–1/2 cups of red lentils.
- 2 tsp. dried sage.
- 7 cups of vegetable broth.
- Mineral sea salt.
- White or fresh cracked pepper.
- cilantro

Preparation:

1. Preheat the oil in a stockpot. Add the onions, then cook for about 5 minutes. Add in the sage and squash. Cook for 5 minutes.

2. Add broth, pepper, lentils, and salt. Cook gradually for 30 minutes on low heat. Pour the mixture using a handheld blender. Garnish with

cilantro.

3. Serve and enjoy.

Nutrition:

- Calories: 323.
- Fat: 7.5g.
- Carbs: 21.4g.
- Protein: 10.1g.

32. Cauliflower Potato Curry

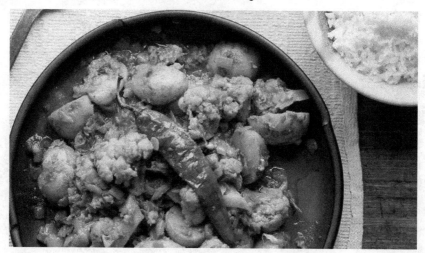

Preparation time: 10 minutes.

Cooking time: 35 minutes.

Servings: 4.

Ingredients:

- 2 tbsps. vegetable oil.
- 1 large chopped onion.
- A large grated piece of ginger.
- 3 finely chopped chive stalks.
- 1/2 tsp. turmeric.
- 1 tsp. ground cumin.
- 1 tsp. curry powder.
- 1 cup of chopped tomatoes.
- 1/2 tsp. sugar.
- 1 florets cauliflower.
- 2 chopped potatoes.
- 1 small halved lengthways green chili.
- A squeeze of Seville orange juice.

- Handful roughly chopped coriander.

Preparation:

1. Add the onion to a greased skillet, then sauté until soft. Add all the spices to the skillet, then stir.

2. Add the cauliflower and potatoes.

3. Sauté for about 5 minutes, then add green chilies, tomatoes, and sugar. Cover, then cook for about 30 minutes.

4. Serve warm with the coriander and Seville orange juice and enjoy.

Nutrition:

- Calories: 332.
- Fat: 7.5g.
- Carbs: 19.4g.
- Protein: 3.1g.

33. Vegetable Bean Curry

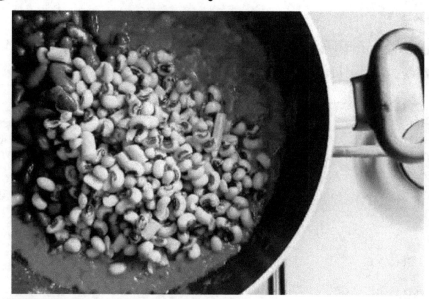

Preparation time: 5 minutes.

Cooking time: 6 hours.

Servings: 8.

Ingredients:

- 1 finely chopped onion.
- 4 chopped chive stalks.
- 3 tsp. coriander powder.
- 1/2 tsp. cinnamon powder.
- 1 tsp. ginger powder.
- 1 tsp. turmeric powder.
- 1/2 tsp. cayenne pepper.
- 2 tbsps. tomato paste.
- 1 tbsp. avocado oil.
- 2 cans, 15 ozs. each, well rinsed and drained lima beans.
- 3 cups of cubed and peeled turnips.
- 3 cups of fresh cauliflower florets.

- 4 medium diced zucchinis.
- 2 medium seeded and chopped tomatoes.
- 2 cups of vegetable broth.
- 1 cup of light coconut milk.
- 1/2 tsp. pepper.
- 1/4 tsp. sea salt.

Preparation:

1. In a slow cooker, preheat the oil, then add all the vegetables. Add in the remaining ingredients, then stir. Cook for about 6 hours at low temperature.

2. Serve warm and enjoy.

Nutrition:

- Calories: 403.
- Fat: 12.5g.
- Carbs: 21.4g.
- Protein: 8.1g.

34. Wild Mushroom Soup

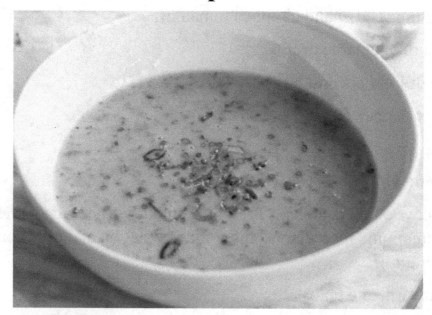

Preparation time: 10 minutes.

Cooking Time: 15 minutes.

Servings: 4.

Ingredients:

- 4 oz. walnut butter.
- 1 chopped shallot.
- 5 oz. chopped portabella mushrooms.
- 5 oz. chopped oyster mushrooms.
- 5 oz. chopped shiitake mushrooms.
- 1 minced chive clove.
- 1/2 tsp. dried thyme.
- 3 cups of alkaline water.
- 1 vegetable bouillon cube.
- 1 cup of coconut cream.
- 1/2 lb. chopped celery root.

- 1 tbsp. white wine vinegar.
- Fresh cilantro.

Preparation:

1. In a cooking pan, melt the butter over medium heat. Add the vegetables into the pan, then sauté until golden brown.

2. Add the remaining ingredients to the pan, then correctly mix it. Boil the mixture. Simmer it for 15 minutes on low heat.

3. Add the cream to the soup, then pour it using a handheld blender. Serve warm with the chopped cilantro as toppings.

Nutrition:

- Calories: 243.
- Fat: 7.5g.
- Carbs: 14.4g.
- Protein: 10.1g.

35. Bok Choy Soup

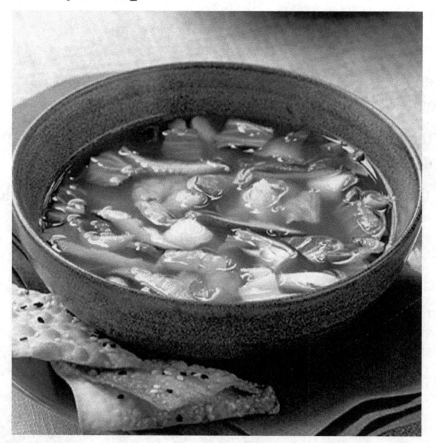

Preparation time: 5 minutes.

Cooking time: 10 minutes.

Servings: 2.

Ingredients:

- 1 cup of chopped bok choy.
- 3 cups of vegetable broth.
- 2 peeled and sliced zucchinis.
- 1/2 cup of cooked hemp seed.
- 1 roughly chopped bunch radish.

Preparation:

1. In a pan, mix the ingredients over moderate heat. Let it simmer, then cook it for about 10 minutes until the vegetables become tender.

2. Serve and enjoy.

Nutrition:

- Calories: 172.
- Fat: 3.5g.
- Carbs: 38.5g.
- Protein: 11.7g.

36. Grilled Vegetable Stack

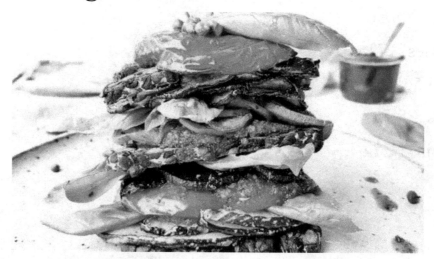

Preparation time: 10 minutes.

Cooking time: 20 minutes.

Servings: 2.

Ingredients:

- 1/2 zucchini, sliced into slices about ¼-inch thick.
- 2 stemmed Portobello mushrooms with the gills removed.
- 1 tsp. divided sea salt.
- 1/2 cup of divided hummus.
- 1 peeled and sliced red onion.
- 1 seeded red bell pepper, sliced lengthwise.
- 1 seeded yellow bell pepper, sliced lengthwise.

Preparation:

1. Adjust the temperature of your broiler or grill. Grill the mushroom caps over coal or gas flame.

2. Add the yellow and red bell peppers, onion, and zucchini for about 20 minutes as you turn it occasionally.

3. Fill the mushroom cap with 1/4 cup of hummus. Top it with some onion, yellow peppers, red, and zucchini. Add salt to season, then set it

aside.

4. Redo the process with the second mushroom cap and the remaining ingredients.

5. Serve and enjoy.

Nutrition:

- Calories: 179.
- Fat: 3.1g.
- Carbs: 15.7g.
- Protein: 3.9g.

37. Date Night Chive Bake

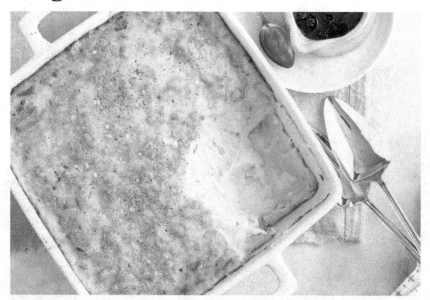

Preparation time: 10 minutes.

Cooking time: 30 minutes.

Servings: 2.

Ingredients:

- 4 peeled and sliced lengthwise zucchinis.
- 1 lb. radish chopped into bite-size pieces.
- 2 tsp. Seville orange zest.
- 3 peeled and chopped chive heads cloves.
- 2 tbsps. coconut oil.
- 1 cup of vegetable broth.
- 1/4 tsp. mustard powder.
- 1 tsp. sea salt.

Preparation:

1. Adjust the temperature of the oven to 400ºF. In a separate bowl, mix all the ingredients.

2. Spread the mixture in a baking pan evenly. Cover the mixture with a piece of aluminum foil, then place it in the oven.

3. Bake the mixture for about 30 minutes as you stir it once halfway through the cooking time.

4. Serve and enjoy.

Nutrition:

- Calories: 270.
- Fat: 15.2g.
- Carbs: 28.1g.
- Protein: 11.6g.

Chapter 13. 30-Day Meal Plan

Day	Breakfast	Lunch	Dinner
1	Alkaline blueberry spelt pancakes	Jackfruit vegetable fry	Veggie medley
2	Crunchy quinoa meal	Alkaline sausage links	Tangy lentil soup
3	Coconut pancakes	Turnip green soup	Vegetable casserole
4	Banana barley porridge	Lentil kale soup	Cauliflower potato curry
5	Zucchini muffins	Mushroom leek soup	Vegetable bean curry
6	Millet porridge	Red lentil squash soup	Grilled vegetable stack
7	Zucchini pancakes	Wild mushroom soup	Date night chive bake
8	Squash hash	Bok Choy soup	Jackfruit vegetable fry
9	Hemp seed porridge	Veggie medley	Alkaline sausage links
10	Alkaline blueberry and strawberry muffins	Tangy lentil soup	Turnip green soup
11	Teff breakfast porridge	Vegetable casserole	Lentil kale soup
12	Breakfast blackberry bars	Cauliflower Potato Curry	Mushroom leek soup
13	Butternut squash bash	Vegetable bean Curry	Red lentil squash soup

	browns		
14	Blueberry spelt flat cakes	Grilled vegetable stack	Wild mushroom soup
15	Breakfast quinoa cereal	Date night chive bake	Bok Choy soup
16	Sweet date quinoa porridge	Jackfruit vegetable fry	Veggie medley
17	Alkaline blueberry Spelt pancakes	Alkaline sausage links	Tangy lentil soup
18	Crunchy quinoa meal	Turnip green soup	Vegetable casserole
19	Coconut pancakes	Lentil kale soup	Cauliflower Potato Curry
20	Banana barley porridge	Mushroom leek soup	Vegetable bean Curry
21	Zucchini muffins	Red lentil squash soup	Grilled vegetable stack
22	Millet porridge.	Wild mushroom soup.	Date night chive bake.
23	Zucchini pancakes	Bok Choy soup	Jackfruit vegetable fry
24	Squash hash	Veggie medley	Jackfruit vegetable fry
25	Hemp seed porridge	Tangy lentil soup	Alkaline sausage links
26	Alkaline blueberry and strawberry muffins	Vegetable casserole	Turnip green soup
27	Teff breakfast porridge	Cauliflower Potato Curry	Lentil kale soup

28	Breakfast blackberry bars	Vegetable bean Curry	Mushroom leek soup
29	Butternut squash Hash browns	Grilled vegetable stack	Red lentil squash soup
30	Blueberry spelt flat cakes	Date night chive bake	Wild mushroom soup

Conclusion

The diet of Dr. Sebi encourages consuming whole, unprocessed, food based on plants. It will support weight reduction if you do eat this way regularly. It depends heavily on taking the pricey vitamins of Dr. Sebi, also is rather rigid, removes essential nutrients, and claims to shift your body to an alkaline condition.

Many healthier foods are more versatile and safer if you're trying to adopt a more plant-based eating trend. Its heavy focus on plant-based ingredients is one feature of the Dr. Sebi diet. The diet allows a significant variety of vegetables and fruits that are rich in minerals, nutrition, vitamins, and plant compounds to be eaten. As a result, your body can have reduced inflammation, and less cell proliferation and defense against multiple illnesses have been linked with diets high in vegetables and berries. In a report, persons who consumed seven or more vegetables and fruit servings each day had a 25%-31% lower risk of heart disease, cancer, and diabetes. Moreover, most people do not consume enough fruit.

The Dr. Sebi diet encourages consuming whole grains high in fiber and good fats, such as seeds, nuts, and plant oils. The reduced incidence of heart failure has been correlated with these foods.

Finally, there are no clear nutrient recommendations for diets that restrict ultra-processed foods correlated with higher overall diet consistency. Though, this diet is weak in nutrition, as grains, soy products, lentils, and animal products are banned. Protein is an essential nutrient needed for healthy muscles, joints, and skin. You are also supposed to buy cell food items from Dr. Sebi, which are vitamins that aim to nourish your cells and cleanse your body.

The "all-inclusive" kit, which includes 20 separate items that are said to cleanse and heal your whole body at the quickest possible rate, is suggested to be bought. Besides this, no specific supplement recommendations are provided. You're supposed to request some supplement that suits your health issues.

For example, the "Bio Ferro" capsules promise to cure liver problems, improve immunity, cleanse the blood, encourage weight loss, help digestive issues, and enhance overall well-being. Furthermore, the medicines don't provide a full list of nutrients or proportions, rendering it impossible to recognize if they can suit everyday needs.

The Benefits from Dr. Sebi's Diet

A plant-based alkaline diet can provide you with these benefits:

- **Weight loss:** a vegan diet has culminated in greater weight loss than other diets that are less stringent. After six months on a plant-based diet, people can lose up to 7.5% of their body weight.

- **Appetite control:** research participants reported that after consuming a plant-based meal comprising of beans and peas, they feel fuller and happier than a meat-related meal.

- **Alter the microbiota:** the word "microbiome" collectively applies to the microorganisms in the stomach, modifying the microbiome. It was observed that a plant-based diet could favorably alter the microbiota, resulting in less disease danger. Confirming this would, however, take further study.

- **Lower risk of disease:** research concluded that a plant-based diet would decrease by 40% the risk of coronary heart disease and by half the risk of developing type 2 diabetes and metabolic syndrome.

In a nutshell, Dr. Sebi's Nutritional Guide Diet inspires people to avoid pre-packaged, processed foods, and eat whole foods, grains. According to research, it has been proven that reducing the intake of pre-packaged processed food and meat quantity improves the nutritional excellence of the general diet in the community.